Opportunities and Challenges for Using Digital Health Applications in Oncology

PROCEEDINGS OF A WORKSHOP

Erin Balogh, Anne Frances Johnson, and Sharyl Nass, *Rapporteurs*

National Cancer Policy Forum

Board on Health Care Services

Health and Medicine Division

and

Forum on Cyber Resilience

Division on Engineering and Physical Sciences

The National Academies of
SCIENCES • ENGINEERING • MEDICINE

THE NATIONAL ACADEMIES PRESS
Washington, DC
www.nap.edu

THE NATIONAL ACADEMIES PRESS   500 Fifth Street, NW   Washington, DC 20001

This activity was supported by Contract No. 200-2011-38807 (Task Order No. 75D30120F00089) and Contract No. HHSN263201800029I (Task Order No. HHSN26300008) with the Centers for Disease Control and Prevention and the National Cancer Institute/National Institutes of Health, respectively, and by the American Association for Cancer Research, American Cancer Society, American College of Radiology, American Society of Clinical Oncology, Association of American Cancer Institutes, Association of Community Cancer Centers, Bristol-Myers Squibb, Cancer Support Community, CEO Roundtable on Cancer, Flatiron Health, Merck, National Comprehensive Cancer Network, National Patient Advocate Foundation, Novartis Oncology, Oncology Nursing Society, Pfizer Inc., Sanofi, and Society for Immunotherapy of Cancer. Any opinions, findings, conclusions, or recommendations expressed in this publication do not necessarily reflect the views of any organization or agency that provided support for the project.

International Standard Book Number-13: 978-0-309-08922-7
International Standard Book Number-10: 0-309-08922-0
Digital Object Identifier: https://doi.org/10.17226/26286

Additional copies of this publication are available from the National Academies Press, 500 Fifth Street, NW, Keck 360, Washington, DC 20001; (800) 624-6242 or (202) 334-3313; http://www.nap.edu.

Copyright 2021 by the National Academy of Sciences. All rights reserved.

Printed in the United States of America

Suggested citation: National Academies of Sciences, Engineering, and Medicine. 2021. *Opportunities and challenges for using digital health applications in oncology: Proceedings of a workshop*. Washington, DC: The National Academies Press. https://doi.org/10.17226/26286.

The National Academies of
SCIENCES · ENGINEERING · MEDICINE

The **National Academy of Sciences** was established in 1863 by an Act of Congress, signed by President Lincoln, as a private, nongovernmental institution to advise the nation on issues related to science and technology. Members are elected by their peers for outstanding contributions to research. Dr. Marcia McNutt is president.

The **National Academy of Engineering** was established in 1964 under the charter of the National Academy of Sciences to bring the practices of engineering to advising the nation. Members are elected by their peers for extraordinary contributions to engineering. Dr. John L. Anderson is president.

The **National Academy of Medicine** (formerly the Institute of Medicine) was established in 1970 under the charter of the National Academy of Sciences to advise the nation on medical and health issues. Members are elected by their peers for distinguished contributions to medicine and health. Dr. Victor J. Dzau is president.

The three Academies work together as the **National Academies of Sciences, Engineering, and Medicine** to provide independent, objective analysis and advice to the nation and conduct other activities to solve complex problems and inform public policy decisions. The National Academies also encourage education and research, recognize outstanding contributions to knowledge, and increase public understanding in matters of science, engineering, and medicine.

Learn more about the National Academies of Sciences, Engineering, and Medicine at **www.nationalacademies.org**.

The National Academies of
SCIENCES · ENGINEERING · MEDICINE

Consensus Study Reports published by the National Academies of Sciences, Engineering, and Medicine document the evidence-based consensus on the study's statement of task by an authoring committee of experts. Reports typically include findings, conclusions, and recommendations based on information gathered by the committee and the committee's deliberations. Each report has been subjected to a rigorous and independent peer-review process and it represents the position of the National Academies on the statement of task.

Proceedings published by the National Academies of Sciences, Engineering, and Medicine chronicle the presentations and discussions at a workshop, symposium, or other event convened by the National Academies. The statements and opinions contained in proceedings are those of the participants and are not endorsed by other participants, the planning committee, or the National Academies.

For information about other products and activities of the National Academies, please visit www.nationalacademies.org/about/whatwedo.

WORKSHOP PLANNING COMMITTEE[1]

LAWRENCE N. SHULMAN (*Chair*), Professor of Medicine, Deputy Director for Clinical Services, and Director, Center for Global Cancer Medicine, Abramson Cancer Center, University of Pennsylvania

KAREN BASEN-ENGQUIST, Annie Laurie Howard Research Distinguished Professor, Professor of Behavioral Science; and Director, Center for Energy Balance in Cancer Prevention and Survivorship, The University of Texas MD Anderson Cancer Center

CATHY J. BRADLEY, David F. and Margaret Turley Grohne Chair for Cancer Prevention and Control Research; Professor and Associate Dean for Research, Colorado School of Public Health; and Deputy Director, University of Colorado Cancer Center

DEBORAH ESTRIN, Associate Dean for Impact and Robert V. Tishman '37 Professor, Computer Science Department, Cornell Tech

LISA KENNEDY SHELDON, Clinical and Scientific Affairs Liaison, Oncology Nursing Society; and Oncology Nurse Practitioner, St. Joseph Hospital

MIA LEVY, Sheba Foundation Director, Rush University Cancer Center; Associate Professor of Medicine, Division of Hematology and Oncology; and System Vice President, Cancer Services, Rush System for Health

J. LEONARD LICHTENFELD, Deputy Chief Medical Officer, American Cancer Society

BRADLEY MALIN, Vice Chair and Professor of Biomedical Informatics, and Professor of Biostatistics and Computer Science, Vanderbilt University Medical Center

DEVEN McGRAW, Chief Regulatory Officer, Ciitizen

NEAL J. MEROPOL, Vice President and Head of Medical and Scientific Affairs, Flatiron Health; and Adjunct Professor, Case Comprehensive Cancer Center

RANDALL A. OYER, Medical Director, Oncology, Ann B. Barshinger Cancer Institute; Medical Director, Cancer Risk Evaluation Program, Penn Medicine Lancaster General Health; and President, Association of Community Cancer Centers

---

[1] The National Academies of Sciences, Engineering, and Medicine's planning committees are solely responsible for organizing the workshop, identifying topics, and choosing speakers. The responsibility for the published Proceedings of a Workshop rests with the workshop rapporteurs and the institution.

Project Staff

ADEGBOYEGA AKINSIKU, Christine Mirzayan Science & Technology Policy Fellow (*from January–April 2020*)
RACHEL AUSTIN, Senior Program Associate
LORI BENJAMIN BRENIG, Research Associate
ANNALEE GONZALES, Administrative Assistant
LYNETTE MILLETT, Director, Forum on Cyber Resilience
ERIN BALOGH, Co-Director, National Cancer Policy Forum
SHARYL NASS, Co-Director, National Cancer Policy Forum, and Senior Director, Board on Health Care Services

NATIONAL CANCER POLICY FORUM[1]

EDWARD J. BENZ, JR. (*Chair*), President and Chief Executive Officer Emeritus, Dana-Farber Cancer Institute; and Richard and Susan Smith Distinguished Professor of Medicine, Genetics and Pediatrics, Harvard Medical School

PETER C. ADAMSON, Global Head, Oncology Development and Pediatric Innovation, Sanofi

GARNET L. ANDERSON, Senior Vice President and Director, Public Health Sciences Division, Fred Hutchinson Cancer Research Center; and Affiliate Professor, Department of Biostatistics, University of Washington

KAREN BASEN-ENGQUIST, Annie Laurie Howard Research Distinguished Professor, Professor of Behavioral Science; and Director, Center for Energy Balance in Cancer Prevention and Survivorship, The University of Texas MD Anderson Cancer Center

SMITA BHATIA, Professor and Vice Chair of Outcomes for Pediatrics; Gay and Bew White Endowed Chair in Pediatric Oncology; Director, Institute for Cancer Outcomes and Survivorship; and Associate Director for Outcomes Research, Comprehensive Cancer Center, The University of Alabama at Birmingham

CHRIS BOSHOFF, Chief Development Officer, Oncology, Global Product Development, Pfizer Inc.

CATHY J. BRADLEY, David F. and Margaret Turley Grohne Chair for Cancer Prevention and Control Research; Professor and Associate Dean for Research, Colorado School of Public Health; and Deputy Director, University of Colorado Cancer Center

OTIS W. BRAWLEY, Bloomberg Distinguished Professor, Department of Epidemiology, Bloomberg School of Public Health, Department of Oncology, School of Medicine, Sidney Kimmel Comprehensive Cancer Center, Johns Hopkins University

CYNTHIA BROGDON, Head, U.S. Oncology Portfolio Strategy, Bristol-Myers Squibb

WILLIAM G. CANCE, Chief Medical and Scientific Officer, American Cancer Society

---

[1] The National Academies of Sciences, Engineering, and Medicine's forums and roundtables do not issue, review, or approve individual documents. The responsibility for the published Proceedings of a Workshop rests with the workshop rapporteurs and the institution.

ROBERT W. CARLSON, Chief Executive Officer, National Comprehensive Cancer Network
CHRISTINA CHAPMAN, Assistant Professor of Radiation Oncology, University of Michigan
GWEN DARIEN, Executive Vice President, Patient Advocacy and Engagement, National Patient Advocate Foundation
NANCY E. DAVIDSON, President and Executive Director, Seattle Cancer Care Alliance; Raisebeck Endowed Chair for Collaborative Research, Senior Vice President, Director, and Professor, Clinical Research Division, Fred Hutchinson Cancer Research Center, and Head, Department of Medicine, Division of Medical Oncology, University of Washington
JAMES H. DOROSHOW, Director, Division of Cancer Treatment and Diagnosis; Deputy Director for Clinical and Translational Research; and Head, Oxidative Signaling and Molecular Therapeutics Group, National Cancer Institute
NICOLE F. DOWLING, Associate Director for Science, Division of Cancer Prevention and Control, Centers for Disease Control and Prevention
SCOT W. EBBINGHAUS, Vice President and Therapeutic Area Head, Oncology Clinical Research, Merck Research Laboratories
KOJO S. J. ELENITOBA-JOHNSON, Professor, Perelman School of Medicine; and Director, Center for Personalized Diagnostics and Division of Precision and Computational Diagnostics, University of Pennsylvania
STANTON L. GERSON, Director, Case Comprehensive Cancer Center; Interim Dean and Senior Vice President, Medical Affairs, School of Medicine; Professor, Department of Medicine and Department of Environmental Health Sciences; Director, National Center for Regenerative Medicine, Case Western Reserve University
JULIE R. GRALOW, Executive Vice President and Chief Medical Officer, American Society of Clinical Oncology
ROY S. HERBST, Ensign Professor of Medicine and Professor of Pharmacology; Director, Center for Thoracic Cancers; Chief of Medical Oncology, Yale Cancer Center and Smilow Cancer Hospital; Associate Cancer Center Director, Translational Science, Yale School of Medicine
HEDVIG HRICAK, Chair, Department of Radiology, Memorial Sloan Kettering Cancer Center

CHANITA HUGHES-HALBERT, Vice Chair for Research and Professor, Department of Preventive Medicine, Associate Director for Cancer Equity, Norris Comprehensive Cancer Center, University of Southern California

MIMI HUIZINGA, Vice President and Head, U.S. Oncology Medical, Novartis Oncology

ROY A. JENSEN, Director, The University of Kansas Cancer Center; William R. Jewell, M.D. Distinguished Masonic Professor, Kansas Masonic Cancer Research Institute; and Immediate Past President, Association of American Cancer Institutes

RANDY A. JONES, Professor of Nursing, Robert Wood Johnson Foundation Nurse Faculty Scholar Alumnus, University of Virginia School of Nursing

BETH Y. KARLAN, Vice Chair, Women's Health Research Professor, Department of Obstetrics and Gynecology, David Geffen School of Medicine; and Director, Cancer Population Genetics, Jonsson Comprehensive Cancer Center, University of California, Los Angeles

SAMIR N. KHLEIF, Director, Jeannie and Tony Loop Immuno-Oncology Lab; and Biomedical Scholar and Professor of Oncology, Georgetown Lombardi Comprehensive Cancer Center, Georgetown University Medical Center

MIA LEVY, Sheba Foundation Director, Rush University Cancer Center; Associate Professor of Medicine, Division of Hematology and Oncology; and System Vice President, Cancer Services, Rush System for Health

SCOTT M. LIPPMAN, Director, Moores Cancer Center; Distinguished Professor of Medicine, Senior Associate Dean, and Associate Vice Chancellor for Cancer Research and Care, and Chugai Pharmaceutical Chair in Cancer, University of California, San Diego

NEAL J. MEROPOL, Vice President and Head of Medical and Scientific Affairs, Flatiron Health; and Adjunct Professor, Case Comprehensive Cancer Center

LARISSA NEKHLYUDOV, Professor of Medicine, Harvard Medical School; Internist, Brigham and Women's Hospital; and Clinical Director, Internal Medicine for Cancer Survivors, Dana-Farber Cancer Institute

RANDALL A. OYER, Medical Director, Oncology, Ann B. Barshinger Cancer Institute; Medical Director, Cancer Risk Evaluation Program, Penn Medicine Lancaster General Health; and President, Association of Community Cancer Centers

CLEO A. SAMUEL-RYALS, Associate Professor of Health Policy and Management, Gillings School of Global Public Health, University of North Carolina at Chapel Hill

RICHARD L. SCHILSKY, Principal Investigator, American Society of Clinical Oncology Targeted Agent and Profiling Utilization Registry (TAPUR^{TM}) Study; and Professor Emeritus, University of Chicago

JULIE SCHNEIDER, Associate Director, Research Strategy and Partnership, Oncology Center of Excellence, Food and Drug Administration

SUSAN M. SCHNEIDER, Associate Professor, Emerita, Duke University School of Nursing

LAWRENCE N. SHULMAN, Professor of Medicine, Deputy Director for Clinical Services, and Director, Center for Global Cancer Medicine, Abramson Cancer Center, University of Pennsylvania

LARA STRAWBRIDGE, Director, Division of Ambulatory Payment Models, Patient Care Models Group, Center for Medicare & Medicaid Innovation, Centers for Medicare & Medicaid Services

GEORGE J. WEINER, C.E. Block Chair of Cancer Research, Professor of Internal Medicine and Pharmaceutical Science, and Director, Holden Comprehensive Cancer Center, The University of Iowa

ROBERT A. WINN, Director, Massey Cancer Center; Senior Associate Dean for Cancer Innovation; Professor, Pulmonary Disease and Critical Care Medicine; and Lipman Chair in Oncology, School of Medicine, Virginia Commonwealth University

PHYLICIA L. WOODS, Executive Director, Cancer Policy Institute, Cancer Support Community

National Cancer Policy Forum Staff

FRANCIS AMANKWAH, Program Officer
RACHEL AUSTIN, Senior Program Assistant
LORI BENJAMIN BRENIG, Research Associate
ANNALEE GONZALES, Administrative Assistant
MICAH WINOGRAD, Senior Finance Business Partner

ERIN BALOGH, Co-Director, National Cancer Policy Forum
SHARYL J. NASS, Co-Director, National Cancer Policy Forum, and Senior Director, Board on Health Care Services

Reviewers

This Proceedings of a Workshop was reviewed in draft form by individuals chosen for their diverse perspectives and technical expertise. The purpose of this independent review is to provide candid and critical comments that will assist the National Academies of Sciences, Engineering, and Medicine in making each published proceedings as sound as possible and to ensure that it meets the institutional standards for quality, objectivity, evidence, and responsiveness to the charge. The review comments and draft manuscript remain confidential to protect the integrity of the process.

We thank the following individuals for their review of this proceedings:

CHRISTOPHER R. COGLE, University of Florida
PAUL KLUETZ, Food and Drug Administration
SUSAN K. PETERSON, The University of Texas MD Anderson Cancer Center
KRISTEN B. ROSATI, Coppersmith Brockelman PLC

Although the reviewers listed above provided many constructive comments and suggestions, they were not asked to endorse the content of the proceedings nor did they see the final draft before its release. The review of this proceedings was overseen by **DANIEL MASYS,** University of Washington. He was responsible for making certain that an independent examination of this proceedings was carried out in accordance with standards of the National Academies and that all review comments were carefully considered. Responsibility for the final content rests entirely with the rapporteurs and the National Academies.

Acknowledgments

Support from the many annual sponsors of the National Academies of Sciences, Engineering, and Medicine's National Cancer Policy Forum is crucial to the work of the forum. Federal sponsors include the Centers for Disease Control and Prevention and the National Cancer Institute/National Institutes of Health. Nonfederal sponsors include the American Association for Cancer Research, American Cancer Society, American College of Radiology, American Society of Clinical Oncology, Association of American Cancer Institutes, Association of Community Cancer Centers, Bristol-Myers Squibb, Cancer Support Community, CEO Roundtable on Cancer, Flatiron Health, Merck, National Comprehensive Cancer Network, National Patient Advocate Foundation, Novartis Oncology, Oncology Nursing Society, Pfizer Inc., Sanofi, and Society for Immunotherapy of Cancer.

The forum wishes to express its gratitude to the expert speakers whose presentations helped further the dialogue on opportunities to advance progress in the effective and safe development, implementation, and use of digital health in oncology research and care. The forum also wishes to thank the members of the planning committee for their work in developing an excellent workshop agenda.

Contents

ACRONYMS AND ABBREVIATIONS … xxi

PROCEEDINGS OF A WORKSHOP … 1
WORKSHOP OVERVIEW … 1
OVERVIEW OF DIGITAL HEALTH APPLICATIONS IN ONCOLOGY … 6
DIGITAL HEALTH TECHNOLOGIES FOR PATIENTS AND CLINICIANS … 13
    Patient-Oriented Technologies, 14
    Clinician-Oriented Technologies, 21
HEALTH DATA ACCESS AND USE … 25
    Leveraging Electronic Health Records and Artificial Intelligence to Improve Cancer Care, 25
    Using Artificial Intelligence to Improve Care Delivery, 27
    Making Data Usable, 28
POLICY CONSIDERATIONS … 32
    Regulatory Considerations, 32
    Legal Considerations, 34
    Payment Models, 37
    Ethical Considerations, 39
REFLECTIONS AND SUGGESTIONS … 42
REFERENCES … 44

APPENDIX A: STATEMENT OF TASK 49
APPENDIX B: WORKSHOP AGENDA 51

Boxes, Figures, and Table

BOXES

1 Suggestions from Individual Workshop Participants to Advance the Appropriate Use of Digital Health Applications in Oncology, 3
2 Examples of the Impact of the COVID-19 Pandemic Discussed by Workshop Participants: Rapid Changes in Cancer Research and Care, 7

FIGURES

1 Outpatient visits at the Rush University Cancer Center at the start of the COVID-19 pandemic, 11
2 Number of clinical trials started annually that include a connected digital product, 15
3 Conventional physician-led symptom monitoring leads to underreporting compared to patient-reported outcomes among patients with cancer, 17
4 A workflow model for implementing electronic patient-reported outcomes in oncology clinical practice, 18

TABLE

1 Availability of Different Types of Data in Electronic Health Records, 31

Acronyms and Abbreviations

AI	artificial intelligence
BRCA	BReast CAncer gene
CDRH	Center for Devices and Radiological Health
CMS	Centers for Medicare & Medicaid Services
CodeX	Common Oncology Data Elements eXtensions
EHR	electronic health record
ENE	extranodal extension
ePRO	electronic patient-reported outcome
FDA	Food and Drug Administration
FHIR	Fast Healthcare Interoperability Resources
GA4GH	Global Alliance for Genomics and Health
GDO	Genetic Discrimination Observatory
HIPAA	Health Insurance Portability and Accountability Act
HITECH Act	Health Information Technology for Economic and Clinical Health Act
mCODE	Minimal Common Oncology Data Elements
ML	machine learning

MSK	Memorial Sloan Kettering
MSKCC	Memorial Sloan Kettering Cancer Center
PRO	patient-reported outcome
PRO-CTCAE™	PRO-Common Terminology Criteria for Adverse Events
PROVE	Patient-Reported Outcomes, Value & Experience
SEER	Surveillance, Epidemiology, and End Results program

Proceedings of a Workshop

WORKSHOP OVERVIEW[1]

Digital health encompasses a broad array of tools and strategies with the goals of advancing research, increasing health care access and quality, and making care more personalized, said Mia Levy, director of the Rush University Cancer Center. Levy described digital health as the convergence of digital technology with health and health care to improve and personalize care delivery, and to enhance patient quality of life. Digital health encompasses health content, digital health interventions, and digital applications, such as communication tools connecting patients and clinicians (e.g., secure email in the patient portal, text, chat, video visit), remote monitoring tools, clinical decision support tools, and systems for exchanging health information. Patient-facing tools, tools for clinicians, and systems to facilitate research and care improvement are all part of this diverse landscape, and each raises unique opportunities and potential challenges.

To examine key policy issues for the effective and safe development, implementation, and use of digital health technologies in oncology research and care, the National Cancer Policy Forum collaborated with the Forum on

---

[1] The planning committee's role was limited to planning the workshop, and the Proceedings of a Workshop was prepared by the workshop rapporteurs as a factual summary of what occurred at the workshop. Statements, recommendations, and opinions expressed are those of the individual presenters and participants, and are not necessarily endorsed or verified by the National Academies of Sciences, Engineering, and Medicine, and they should not be construed as reflecting any group consensus.

Cyber Resilience to hold a virtual workshop, Opportunities and Challenges for Using Digital Health Applications in Oncology, on July 13–14, 2020. The workshop convened a broad group of experts, including clinicians and researchers; patient advocates; and representatives of federal agencies, health professional societies, health care organizations, insurers, and the pharmaceutical and health technology industries. Many workshop speakers said that the opportunities presented by digital health tools are particularly compelling for oncology; however, capitalizing on these opportunities necessitates careful attention to the design, implementation, and use of digital health technologies.

Lawrence Shulman, deputy director for clinical services at the Abramson Cancer Center at the University of Pennsylvania, and Fred Schneider, professor of computer science at Cornell University, outlined the goals of the workshop. By convening individuals representing a broad range of expertise, the intent of the workshop was to highlight examples of digital health tools; provide a forum to discuss ethical, regulatory, security, governance, and payment considerations; and to discuss needs and opportunities for moving the field forward. While the workshop was conceptualized prior to the COVID-19 pandemic, the workshop also provided an opportunity to reflect on ways in which the pandemic and its response have catalyzed the uptake of digital health technologies, both in oncology and throughout health care and biomedical research.

This Proceedings of a Workshop summarizes the issues that were discussed at the workshop and highlights suggestions from individual participants, which are included throughout the proceedings and summarized in Box 1. Appendix A includes the Statement of Task for the workshop. The workshop agenda is provided in Appendix B. Speakers' presentations and the workshop webcast have been archived online.[2]

It was not possible for this workshop to provide a comprehensive overview of all digital health applications with potential relevance to oncology care and research. For this reason, workshop discussions focused on four main themes:

1. The promises and pitfalls of digital oncology tools across the spectrum of cancer research and care;
2. Financial, regulatory, ethical, and legal considerations for the implementation and use of digital health tools;
3. Challenges and opportunities for leveraging digital health to improve cancer care; and
4. The COVID-19 pandemic as a proving ground—and accelerator—of digital health.

---

[2] See https://www.nationalacademies.org/event/07-13-2020/opportunities-and-challenges-for-using-digital-health-applications-in-oncology-a-workshop (accessed September 8, 2020).

BOX 1
Suggestions from Individual Workshop Participants to Advance the Appropriate Use of Digital Health Applications in Oncology

Maintaining High-Quality, Evidence-Based, Patient-Centered Care
- Rigorously study the effectiveness of digital health applications to inform best practices for their use in oncology. (Levy, Parikh, Peterson, Shulman)
- Leverage the momentum generated by changes implemented in response to the COVID-19 pandemic to facilitate and sustain broad adoption of digital health technologies that improve cancer care and cancer research. (Shulman)
- Use validated electronic patient-reported outcomes where possible to enhance patient–clinician communication and to improve the quality and efficiency of care. (Basch, Kluetz, Pusic, Takvorian)
- Ensure that telehealth visits maintain the equivalent standard of care that is provided with in-person clinic visits, and that clinicians adequately document a telehealth visit in the patient's electronic health record (EHR). (Belmont)
- Engage patients and clinicians throughout the design, implementation, and use of digital health tools. (Anderson, Campbell, Meropol, Peterson, Shulman)

Addressing Barriers to the Adoption of Digital Health Tools
- Establish reimbursement models and provide economic incentives to encourage adoption of effective digital health tools. (Campbell, Levy, Peterson)
- Evaluate how digital health tools affect the quality and efficiency of care delivery and the impact on patient outcomes to inform appropriate reimbursement models. (Bradley, Strawbridge)
- Integrate digital health into clinical workflows, infrastructure, staffing, and training for effective implementation. (Peterson)
- Clearly communicate with patients about the role of digital health in their care and how their data will be used. (Basch, McGraw, Peterson)
- Recognize and address potential challenges in patient access to digital health tools (e.g., digital literacy, access to devices and Internet service). (Levy, Peterson)

continued

> **BOX 1 Continued**
>
> **Enhancing Research and Regulatory Review**
> - Rigorously study the utility of digital health applications in clinical research and apply the results to establish best practices for their use. (Kluetz)
> - Use telehealth and digital tools to broaden the geographic reach of and patient representation in clinical trials. (Shah, Shulman)
> - Capitalize on opportunities to draw on real-world data (such as EHRs) to complement clinical trials research to fill evidence gaps and improve care delivery. (Campbell, Kluetz, Kurian, Meropol, Shulman)
> - Maintain a strong commitment to science and patient safety while expediting review processes and the incorporation of digital health into clinical trials in the context of the COVID-19 pandemic. (Abernethy, Shah)
>
> **Ensuring the Quality of Data and Digital Health Tools**
> - Critically examine the types and quality of real-world data that are available for use by researchers, clinicians, and patients, and assess which methods are most appropriate to capture and present data to the intended users. (Kluetz, Meropol)
> - Establish common data elements and data standards to enable interoperability and data sharing. (Bertagnolli, Meropol)
> - Facilitate responsible data sharing through appropriate data governance and regulation that ensures ethical data use, data security, and patient privacy. (Joly, Kass, Rosati)
> - Ensure that digital health technologies are validated and of high quality when used in clinical research and care. (Kluetz, Peterson)
> - Ensure that the development pathway for an algorithm-based digital health tool includes testing across a broad range of circumstances and populations to support the generalizability of the digital health tool. (Fuchs)

Participants discussed myriad opportunities for using digital health tools to enhance cancer care by expanding access to high-quality care; using scarce medical resources more efficiently; improving patient–clinician communication; and enabling patients to safely and effectively manage more aspects of their care at home, especially during the ongoing pandemic. However, many participants cautioned that digital health is not a panacea. Many participants stressed the need to critically evaluate digital health development and imple-

- Establish benchmarks to assess and improve algorithm performance for medical image analysis. (Aneja, Fuchs)

Protecting Patients
- Establish enforceable patient rights when incorporating patient data into digital health systems. (Downing, Rosati)
- Establish clear legal responsibilities for all entities that interact with patient data, including health care providers and payers, as well as third-party application developers or data aggregators. (Downing, Rosati)
- Avoid exacerbation of existing health disparities by validating digital health technologies for use by diverse populations and minimizing the potential for biased results. (Ferryman, Shulman)
- Communicate clearly the purpose and potential benefits and risks of data aggregation when requesting patient consent for data access and use. (Kass, Shulman)
- Keep promises made to patients regarding the protection of their health data, including adequate measures for data security and patient privacy; if a data breach occurs, provide an appropriate remedy. (Kass, McGraw)
- Ensure that medical liability laws adapt to the new health technology landscape, including circumstances when using a digital health tool contributes to a medical error. (Belmont)
- Explore community-based models for data collection, sharing, and use, particularly for marginalized communities. (Ferryman)

NOTE: This list is the rapporteurs' summary of points made by the individual speakers identified, and the statements have not been endorsed or verified by the National Academies of Sciences, Engineering, and Medicine. They are not intended to reflect a consensus among workshop participants.

mentation and rigorously measure impact. Like any technology or medical tool, digital health tools pose potential risks for the safety and privacy of patients and the security of health data; they also have associated ethical, legal, and financial ramifications. While they offer many exciting possibilities to improve cancer care, several participants noted, these technologies also have the potential to create access barriers and exacerbate disparities unless they are carefully designed, implemented, and evaluated.

Several speakers noted that the successful adoption of digital health tools will also depend on the regulatory and reimbursement environment. Differing—and sometimes conflicting—incentives among digital health developers, regulatory agencies, insurers, health care organizations, clinicians, and patients can complicate the development and implementation pathway for digital health technologies. For many tools, it is unclear how digital health will fit within existing clinical workflows. Similarly, the legal and regulatory frameworks for digital health tools vary widely depending on the type of tool and how it is used in research and care contexts; and in some instances, the regulatory and legal frameworks are still in development or may need to evolve to accommodate how digital health tools are being leveraged in cancer care and cancer research.

Many speakers noted that the COVID-19 pandemic has emerged as an unexpected proving ground and accelerator for digital health (see Box 2). In response to the temporary shutdown of routine in-person patient care, health care delivery practices changed rapidly and many health systems and clinical trials investigators swiftly adopted telehealth and other technologies in order to deliver care or advance cancer research while minimizing face-to-face contact (see Figure 1). Several participants pointed to the need to assess the effects of these changes.

Several speakers noted that it remains unclear which of the recent changes in practice and policy will persist in the long term, and which are only temporary. Several participants posited that the oncology and digital health communities have much to gain by gleaning lessons from the pandemic in order to redesign clinical research and care delivery. Moving forward, many participants urged rigorous evaluation of how digital health tools affect patient outcomes, the delivery of cancer care, and the conduct of clinical research. While the field grapples with the many important policy, financial, security, and ethical considerations around the development and adoption of digital health technologies, many participants stressed the importance of maintaining focus on the central goal: delivering high-quality, patient-centered cancer care.

OVERVIEW OF DIGITAL HEALTH APPLICATIONS IN ONCOLOGY

While digital health tools are being implemented across many settings of care and disease areas, Shulman noted that the oncology setting presents unique considerations and potential benefits. The cancer care continuum spans prevention and early detection; diagnosis; cancer treatment, involving an array of diverse and complex treatment options (including clinical trials); palliative care; survivorship care, which can take place over many years; and end-of-life care. To realize the potential benefits of digital health tools through-

> **BOX 2**
> **Examples of the Impact of the COVID-19 Pandemic Discussed by Workshop Participants: Rapid Changes in Cancer Research and Care**
>
> Although this workshop was conceptualized prior to the emergence of the COVID-19 pandemic, its timing in the first months of the pandemic offered an unexpected opportunity to reflect on how the pandemic affected cancer care and research. Many workshop speakers discussed the drastic changes—including the swift adoption of digital health technologies—implemented across the country. "COVID-19 may now serve as a catalyst for transforming cancer care and research as we know it, and driving this transformation will be digital health," said Anand Shah, deputy commissioner for Medical and Scientific Affairs for the Food and Drug Administration (FDA).
>
> **Shifts in Care Delivery**
> The COVID-19 pandemic forced clinical practices and health systems to pivot toward virtual patient interactions, often in a matter of days or weeks. "We have seen many new trends in digital health across the cancer continuum for several years, but the recent coronavirus pandemic has really accelerated our digital health adoption in the United States," said Mia Levy, director of the Rush University Cancer Center. Workshop participants reported that digital tools are increasingly being used in clinical settings to create touchless workflows, allowing, for example, patients to check in for appointments on their own mobile devices. At home, digital health technologies have enabled patients to interact with clinicians directly via telephone, online chat, and video telehealth visits; use remote monitoring tools such as patient-reported outcomes and biosensors to feed data to their health care team; and download health data from various sources onto personal devices.
>
> **Shifts in Clinical Trials and Evaluations of Novel Therapies**
> Shah noted that many clinical trials in oncology have been affected by the pandemic: Patient enrollment slowed, and investigators are unsure how the COVID-19 pandemic will affect data collection and trial completion (Upadhaya et al., 2020). Shah said that FDA has embraced the full extent of its regulatory flexibilities and adopted new approaches to enable the agency to deliver very rapid advice and review during the pandemic, including streamlined
>
> *continued*

BOX 2 Continued

processes and operations for developers and scientists to send in inquiries and requests, and supporting guidance for clinicians and researchers who submit emergency requests to use investigational products for individual patients.

Shah described several changes made by FDA to facilitate the conduct of clinical trials during the pandemic. First, FDA-issued guidance encouraging use of telemedicine or other tools in clinical trials to reduce the risk of COVID-19 exposure associated with in-person clinic visits. Shah noted that this is especially important for patients with cancer, who are likely to be immunocompromised. Second, FDA allowed for expanded use of noninvasive devices, such as spirometers and blood pressure monitors, for remote patient monitoring. Third, FDA is expanding patient access to investigational products and working to identify and address potential cancer drug shortages. In addition, a new program, Patient Voice,[a] will collate patient-reported symptom data collected from previous clinical trials of cancer therapies that have since been approved by FDA. "The clear attention and focus on technologies to reduce [in-person] visits, enable data collection, and ensure continuity in patient communication and care highlight the growing importance of digital health in oncology," Shah said.

FDA has also issued guidance documents for conducting virtual scientific review meetings and facilitating expanded access to digital health interventions. FDA's Oncology Center of Excellence, for example, used virtual meetings to approve 8 new molecular entities and 23 new indications. Throughout these changes, Shah stressed that FDA has maintained its commitment to science, data, and patient safety. "Expediting development is important, but it is also critical during a public health emergency that we do everything we can to ensure patient safety," he said.

Challenges Encountered

The COVID-19 pandemic has also highlighted challenges to the implementation of digital health in oncology. Levy said that her cancer center has encountered inequities in access to digital health. Not all patients have video capability, Internet access, sufficient data plans for using their mobile devices for telemedicine appointments, or the digital literacy needed to benefit from the increasing availability of telehealth. Virtual interactions can also limit a clinician's ability to conduct a full physical exam and forge personal connections with patients. She said the urgency of telehealth deployment during the pandemic resulted in a rush to implement and train the workforce to use these tools. Levy added that the pandemic has also demonstrated the need for scalable home-based solutions for blood collection and infusion administration. In addition to reducing the risks of exposure, moving more care into the home could alleviate burdens for patients, such as the time and transportation required to travel to appointments, even beyond the pandemic.

The pandemic has also underscored the importance of well-developed systems for data collection and sharing. Shulman stressed that real-time data are critical to understanding the effects of COVID-19 disease in patients with cancer, as well as the safety and effectiveness of telemedicine and other changes to health care experienced during the pandemic. "We need data and we need it fast, and the pandemic exposed our deficiencies in data," Shulman said. Paul Kluetz, deputy director of FDA's Oncology Center of Excellence, stressed the value of real-world aggregated data sources, in addition to clinical trials data. He noted that FDA is collaborating with data collection organizations and the COVID-19 Evidence Accelerator[b] program to understand how patients with cancer are affected by COVID-19.

Looking Ahead

Many workshop participants noted that COVID-19-related changes to health care delivery and the conduct of clinical trials were implemented remarkably quickly. Levy identified three factors that facilitated the rapid implementation of telehealth: Congressional approval of emergency use and removal of the rural-only restriction of the Centers for Medicaid & Medicare Services (CMS), state governments' emergency declarations that required telehealth payment equity, and FDA's guidance clarifying the acceptability of remote assessments for research purposes, where appropriate. However, she noted that some reimbursement regulations that established parity between telehealth and in-person care are set to expire. "In order for telehealth to really continue to thrive and succeed in the United States, we are going to need to sustain these policies and make them more robust so that they can be durable," Levy said.

Looking forward, Shah suggested that increased use of digital enrollment and remote assessment tools could decentralize cancer clinical trials to enable more patients to participate in those trials. He added that decentralization could also facilitate the involvement of more diverse, representative populations in clinical trials. Kluetz encouraged evaluation of data from clinical trials that deployed a hybrid decentralized approach during the COVID-19 pandemic to help determine which remote assessment tools work best and to inform clinical cancer research going forward. Similarly, Levy urged evaluations of the effec-

continued

> **BOX 2 Continued**
>
> tiveness of telehealth visits, adding that demonstrated benefit on patient outcomes can help to overcome adoption challenges. In addition, Shah said the use of new digital health tools is an opportunity to study different approaches to study design, data collection, and monitoring, and may also help investigators aggregate and integrate data to better characterize a patient's experience while participating in a clinical trial.
>
> Shulman noted that medicine as a field is generally slow to change. Unlike industries such as financial services, medicine has been late to digitization, and before the COVID-19 pandemic, was, for the most part, still delivered in person during the work week. "Change is hard, but this is our opportunity to carry forward the good that we've learned during the pandemic."
>
> ---
>
> [a] See https://www.fda.gov/about-fda/oncology-center-excellence/project-patient-voice (accessed May 24, 2021).
> [b] See https://evidenceaccelerator.org (accessed May 24, 2021).

out the cancer care continuum, Shulman stated, "We need to be much more creative and aggressive in the use of digital technology." At the same time, he cautioned, technologies and artificial intelligence (AI) tools such as chatbots or diagnostic algorithms can never fully replace human care; their role is to augment and inform clinical decision making.

Shulman, Levy, and several other participants emphasized the importance of ensuring that digital health tools are safe and meaningful for patients and helpful for clinicians, can improve patient outcomes, and are appropriately reimbursed. Levy suggested measuring the effectiveness of digital health interventions using patient outcomes data, such as treatment adherence, avoidance or early warning of adverse events, disease control, and survival. In addition, patient-focused outcomes could include convenience and increased knowledge; health system–level outcomes could include the effects on readmission rates, hospital length of stay, cost avoidance, or efficiency. Levy pointed to a web-based symptom monitoring intervention that improved survival and reduced health care costs for patients with lung cancer (Denis et al., 2019).

A number of participants noted that there are many challenges to the adoption of digital health interventions. One challenge is the broad range of participants involved in the digital health ecosystem, including patients and their families, clinicians, health systems and clinical practices, insurers,

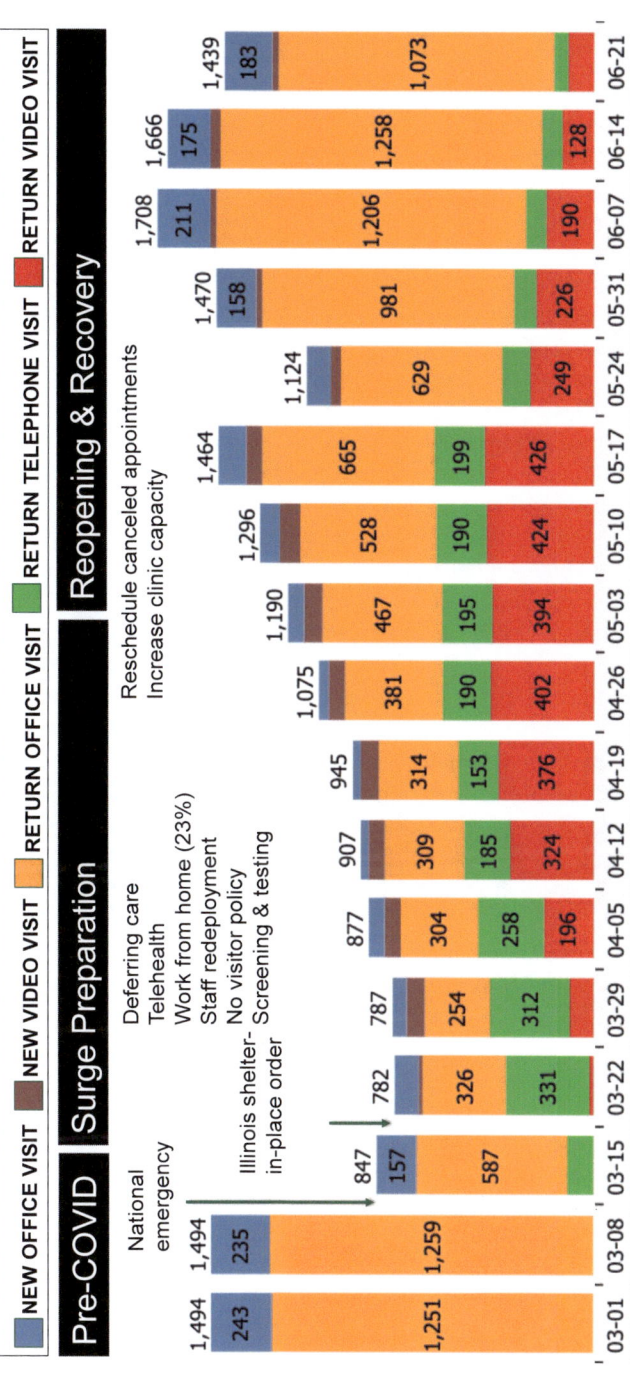

FIGURE 1 Outpatient visits at the Rush University Cancer Center at the start of the COVID-19 pandemic. The Center saw a rapid increase in telephone and video-based visits during the first 3 months of the pandemic.
SOURCE: Levy presentation, July 13, 2020.

and regulators, as well as researchers and vendors who develop and disseminate digital health tools. Because each participant involved in the digital health ecosystem may have differing needs and incentives for digital health tools, Levy said it can be difficult to define who is the customer, what is the value, and who should pay for any particular intervention. She added that digital health interventions are unlikely to be adopted unless participants' financial incentives are aligned and there is a clear and sustainable reimbursement pathway. She noted that in response to the COVID-19 pandemic, insurers implemented reimbursement parity for telemedicine—meaning that clinical visits that are conducted using telehealth are reimbursed at the same financial rate as face-to-face patient encounters. In response to the COVID-19 pandemic, many states also suspended state licensure requirements, which can present another barrier to widespread implementation of telemedicine. While a physician is permitted to treat a patient who lives out of state if the patient travels to the physician's office, state licensure often prevents telemedicine visits with the same patient. However, Levy speculated that these changes are likely temporary, and that achieving a permanent reimbursement strategy for telehealth and other digital health tools, and the regulatory framework to support it, will likely require additional policy action.

Levy said other challenges include: uncertainty regarding how digital health tools will be regulated (NASEM, 2019); limits on how these tools can be used in clinical research; a lack of data standardization; poor integration of digital health tools (with the electronic health record [EHR], for example); and oversight challenges, especially when third-party vendors who handle patient data are not subject to the regulations promulgated under the Health Insurance Portability and Accountability Act (HIPAA).[3] Levy added that another major challenge—especially in regard to ensuring equitable access to digital health tools—is uneven access to the Internet or electronic devices among patients.

Using new digital health tools also requires staff training and adjustments to clinical workflow. Levy noted that it is helpful to rehearse how a new digital health tool will be used in clinical practice, prior to its implementation in patient care. She added that there can be advantages and disadvantages to digital health tools: Some tools may be challenging to integrate into existing workflows, but they may also offer the potential for improvements to patient care, clinician experience, or practice efficiency. If a telemedicine visit is recorded, for example, it could potentially replace or shorten the time it takes clinicians to complete clinical documentation, thereby reducing a clinician's

---

[3] For more information, see https://www.hhs.gov/hipaa/index.html (accessed May 27, 2021).

workload, Levy suggested. In addition, patient-reported outcomes (PROs)[4] are a key part of cancer care and integral to many digital health tools, yet Levy described challenges with integrating them into the EHRs. It can be difficult to develop questions to meet every possible clinical scenario, and the relevance of particular questions may vary substantially depending on a patient's cancer type, disease stage, and type of cancer therapy. She added that most digital tools are highly adaptable, and as a result, differences in PRO configuration and workforce training between institutions hamper the ability to standardize across EHRs. Despite these limitations, Levy suggested that electronic patient-reported outcomes (ePROs) and remote patient monitoring are ripe for more widespread implementation. Shulman suggested an incremental approach to improve adoption of PROs. He noted that integration could be prioritized within certain areas of care that present clear opportunities for patient input, such as patient counseling. In this context and throughout digital health, he urged a scientific approach to identify effective strategies, focus on patient benefit, and build communal will to facilitate progress. Health care "providers, regulators, payers, and patients really need to come together and facilitate change, and any of those groups could be a major deterrent from taking advantage of new opportunities to provide better, more efficient, more effective care," Shulman said. Levy added that successful implementation of digital health tools will require foundational layers of leadership, governance, investment, and infrastructure.

DIGITAL HEALTH TECHNOLOGIES FOR PATIENTS AND CLINICIANS

Several workshop participants shared their experiences with developing, implementing, and evaluating digital health tools across a wide range of uses and settings in oncology.[5]

_____

[4] Patient-reported outcomes are "information about a patient's health that comes directly from the patient. Examples of patient-reported outcomes include a patient's description of their symptoms, their satisfaction with care, and how a disease or treatment affects their physical, mental, emotional, spiritual, and social well-being. In clinical trials, patient-reported outcomes may provide information about the side effects of the new treatment being studied." See https://www.cancer.gov/publications/dictionaries/cancer-terms/def/patient-reported-outcome (access May 26, 2021).

[5] Additional National Academies publications have discussed digital health tools, such as *Improving Cancer Diagnosis and Care: Clinical Application of Computational Methods in Precision Oncology: Proceedings of a Workshop* (NASEM, 2019; Panagiotou et al., 2020), and *The Role of Digital Health Technologies in Drug Development: Proceedings of a Workshop* (NASEM, 2020b).

Patient-Oriented Technologies

Susan K. Peterson, professor at The University of Texas MD Anderson Cancer Center, said that there is a wide variety of patient-oriented digital health technologies, from home blood pressure or physical activity monitors to AI-based chatbots and large-scale data aggregators. Workshop speakers discussed the use of digital health tools for remote monitoring, collection of PROs, and improved patient access to their health data.

Remote Monitoring Technologies

Peterson discussed the use of wearable, mobile, and other remote monitoring technologies in cancer care and cancer research. She noted that remote monitoring technologies share key characteristics: They collect health-related information with potential clinical utility; they are consumer-oriented and require minimal clinician involvement; they include a sensor and software component; and they are portable. These technologies can help clinicians identify when interventions may be needed to prevent or mitigate health problems. Facilitated by continuous, passive data collection, these devices can also overcome barriers that commonly impede traditional data collection efforts, such as the need for active self-reporting or travel to clinical sites to capture this information, Peterson said. Other advantages of remote monitoring devices include the ability to assess key physiological and behavioral outcomes that may otherwise be difficult to capture, and particularly during the COVID-19 pandemic, the potential to minimize in-person clinic visits, Peterson noted.

Peterson said that remote monitoring applications are becoming increasingly integrated into clinical trials (see Figure 2). She noted that clinical trials that include remote technologies typically have one or more of the following goals: to validate device functionality, to test clinical feasibility, to capture trial endpoint data, or to evaluate the impact of the digital health intervention. However, she noted that their use in oncology trials has lagged behind their adoption in other areas of medicine. To advance the use of mobile and wearable technology in oncology clinical trials, Peterson said it is important to prioritize examination of their feasibility, validity, and clinical utility as well as patient and clinician acceptance of the technology.

In cancer, these devices are often used to measure physical activity, which has been associated with reduced hospitalizations, fewer adverse events, and improved survival (Beg et al., 2017; Gresham et al., 2018). Connected devices have also demonstrated usefulness for monitoring PROs in patients with gynecologic cancers, advanced gastrointestinal cancers, and head and neck cancers (Innominato et al., 2018; Peterson et al., 2013; Wright et al., 2018). They have been used to estimate patient performance status, a widely used measure of

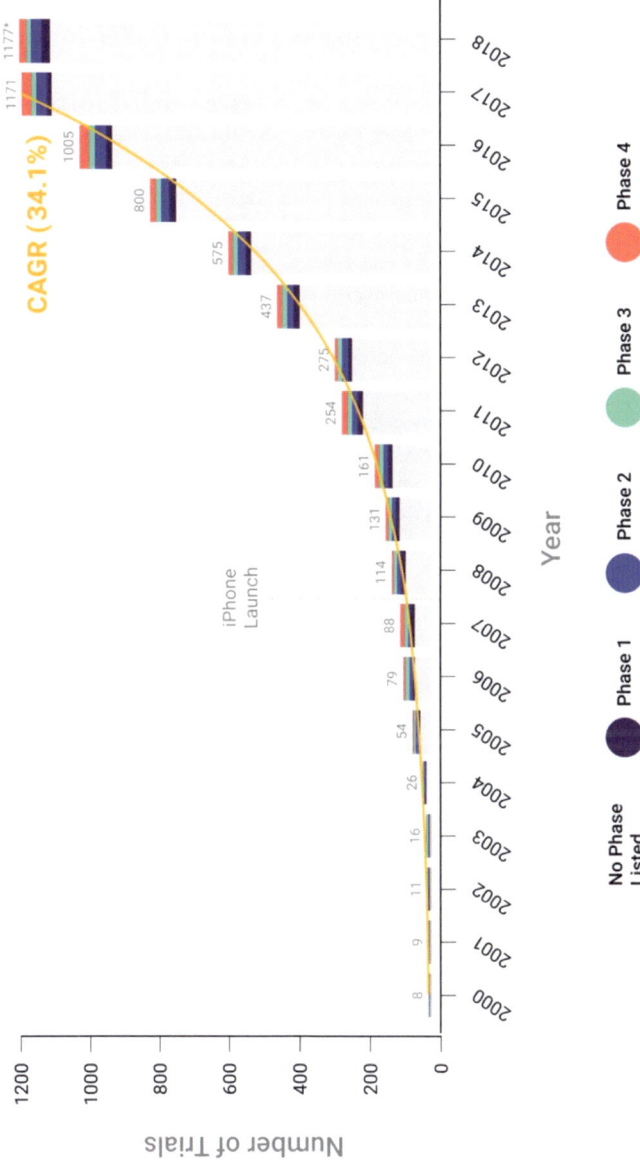

FIGURE 2 Number of clinical trials started annually that include a connected digital product.
NOTES: * 2018 data may be incomplete due to delays by trial sponsors in submitting registration to ClinicalTrials.gov. 2018 trials are not included in the CAGR calculation. CAGR = compound annual growth rate.
SOURCES: Peterson presentation, July 13, 2020; Marra et al., 2020.

physical functioning and overall well-being, as well as to monitor and guide patient care at home. Peterson noted that patient acceptance of these devices is generally high, with many patients reporting that these devices added value to their cancer care. However, she noted that some patients have expressed concern about reduced clinician contact, underscoring the need to offer personal outreach to maintain engagement (Tran et al., 2019).

Looking forward, Peterson said it will be important to build the evidence base for these technologies in oncology to promote their use along the entire continuum of cancer care. She urged the development of infrastructure to support their implementation in diverse populations, particularly among underserved individuals. Peterson noted that health equity challenges—such as disparities in patient access to cancer care, varying digital health literacy rates, and inadequate resources among some health systems—need to be addressed in order to avoid inadvertently exacerbating existing health disparities when implementing digital health tools. In addition, she said financial costs are a key barrier to implementation, so it is imperative for developers to establish a clear business case and reimbursement model, in addition to integrating the tool within existing workflows and staff training. Finally, she noted that it is critical to incentivize the creation of a connected digital ecosystem with interoperable components and open interfaces to further accelerate innovation.

Patient-Reported Outcomes

Several speakers—including Samuel Takvorian, medical oncologist and professor at the University of Pennsylvania Perelman School of Medicine; Andrea Pusic, professor of surgery at Harvard University and chief of plastic and reconstructive surgery at Brigham and Women's Hospital; and Ethan Basch, professor and chief of oncology at the University of North Carolina at Chapel Hill—discussed the collection of PROs in patient-facing digital health applications.

Basch said symptom monitoring is an essential component of cancer care, both to alleviate patients' discomfort and to reduce the risk for complications. Conventional clinician-led symptom monitoring can lead to underreporting of patients' symptoms compared to PROs, said Basch, due to a combination of factors, including limited time in the clinical visit, communication challenges, and human psychology (Basch, 2010) (see Figure 3). PROs provide direct patient reporting on information such as level of pain, physical functioning, and quality of life.

Basch described an ePRO workflow his team developed to support symptom monitoring (see Figure 4). In this closed-loop system, patients receive a prompt via smartphone or telephone, self-report their symptoms, and are referred to a care team member as needed. The system was associated with

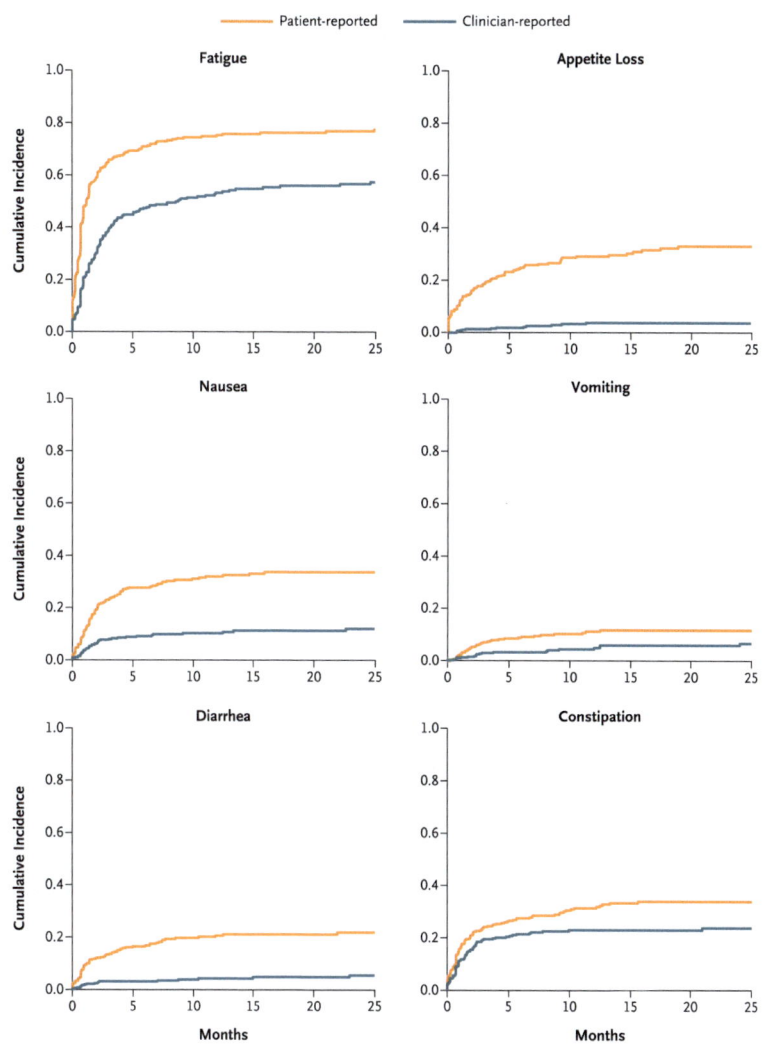

FIGURE 3 Conventional physician-led symptom monitoring (blue line) leads to underreporting compared to patient-reported outcomes (orange line) among patients with cancer.
SOURCES: Basch presentation, July 13, 2020; Basch, 2010.

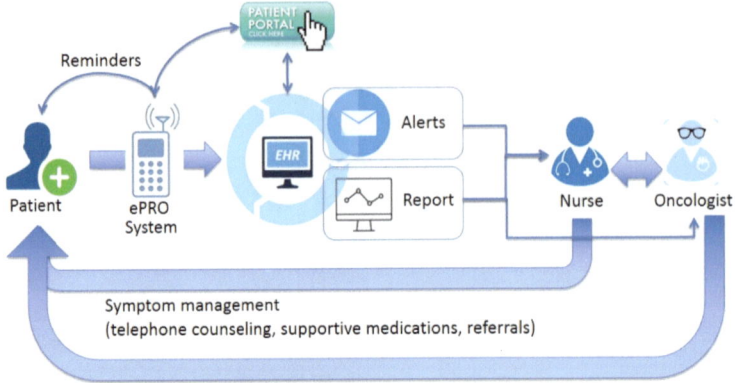

FIGURE 4 A workflow model for implementing electronic patient-reported outcomes in oncology clinical practice.
NOTE: EHR = electronic health record; ePRO = electronic patient-reported outcome.
SOURCE: Basch presentation, July 13, 2020.

improved quality of life, fewer emergency room visits, and longer median overall survival (Barbera et al., 2019; Basch et al., 2016, 2017; Denis et al., 2019). Despite its benefits and an overall positive perception of the ePRO platform among patients and the care team, adoption has been slow, which Basch attributes to the lack of a clear business model to cover its costs. Implementation also requires that clinicians be open to additional workforce training and alterations to existing workflows. To increase ePRO use in oncology, Basch suggested Medicare and private payers should fully reimburse ePRO costs for symptom monitoring. In addition, he said ePROs could be adopted as a performance evaluation measure and included with best practices to ensure sufficient training, full engagement, and compliance monitoring.

Takvorian described Penny, a chatbot used within the University of Pennsylvania health system for oncology symptom management and medication adherence. Penny was built in response to several trends in cancer care: a shift of cancer care from the hospital setting to outpatient clinical practice and in the home, as well as an increase in the use of oral cancer therapies. Takvorian noted that while these trends can be beneficial for patients with cancer, they also transfer much of the responsibility for managing side effects, monitoring symptoms, and following treatment plans onto patients and their caregivers.

Interviews showed that patients preferred asynchronous, mobile-based engagement, so Takvorian's team developed Penny as a smartphone text-messaging program that delivers feedback, based on consensus-based symptom management pathways, directly to patients. Penny uses natural-language processing to respond conversationally to patient-reported symptoms, provide real-time medication instructions, and offer motivational feedback and support. Takvorian added that Penny integrates with the health system's EHR. Penny's adaptive rules engine can analyze patients' reported symptoms and suggest self-management of low-grade symptoms or triage higher-grade symptoms to a clinician. During development, clinicians reviewed patient–bot conversations to make adjustments to the machine learning (ML) model. In a pilot study, Penny demonstrated high participant satisfaction and accurate triaging. Use of the system was also associated with improved medication adherence, reduced clinic call volumes, and fewer emergency department visits. Deborah Estrin, associate dean and professor at Cornell Tech, asked about the ramifications of Penny's human-like characteristics. Takvorian responded that Penny's human feel is critical to its success and has elevated patient engagement, at least anecdotally. He added that empathy is a critical component that requires rigorous study and evaluation.

Pusic described two patient-facing digital applications: the Memorial Sloan Kettering (MSK) Recovery Tracker,[6] and imPROVE, an application for patients with breast cancer. The MSK Recovery Tracker was developed to improve home monitoring and care for patients recovering from surgery. The mobile-based digital application asks patients 11 standard postsurgical questions daily. An algorithm, developed with a combination of clinician input and ML training data, analyzes the responses to identify patients who may need additional follow-up care. After implementating the tracker, Pusic said unnecessary urgent care visits were reduced by 30 percent. Phone calls to nursing staff increased substantially; to reduce the call burden, the team added a feedback feature, which provided patients with a better understanding of which symptoms were considered normal, versus those that may need to be evaluated by their care team. This feedback also enabled care teams to track how patients were recovering and estimate their recovery trajectories. Preliminary analyses from a randomized clinical trial of more than 2,500 patients found that those who used the Recovery Tracker reported less anxiety and a greater sense of connection with their care team. In addition, nursing staff were handling 0.4 fewer nursing calls per patient, which Pusic said was a meaningful reduction given that the center performs more than 10,000 surgeries per year.

Through the Patient-Reported Outcomes, Value & Experience (PROVE) Center at Brigham and Women's Hospital, Pusic and her team are building imPROVE, a breast cancer surgery recovery application similar to the Recovery Tracker but with added emphasis on cancer survivorship care.

---

[6] See https://www.mskcc.org/cancer-care/patient-education/mymsk-recovery-tracker (accessed May 27, 2021).

imPROVE provides tailored feedback, maintains care team connections, and delivers resources to improve patient outcomes. Douglas Peterson, professor at University of Connecticut Health, asked if these telehealth algorithms could be tailored to address a patient's level of health literacy, language, or culture. Pusic said that while further work is needed, her hope is that imPROVE can be adapted across many populations and settings of care, particularly in locations without access to specialized oncology care.

Where possible, Kluetz encouraged developers to use rigorously developed assessment tools that would be appropriate for use in clinical trials, such as the PRO version of the Common Terminology Criteria for Adverse Events[7] (PRO-CTCAE™), when incorporating PROs into digital health tools for routine clinical care. He noted that high-quality ePRO assessments in clinical care can generate a robust stream of structured real-world data that could inform cancer therapy development, pharmacovigilance, and optimal care strategies for patients with cancer. He added that better characterization of the relationship between symptoms and functional outcomes can better support patients' decisions about treatment.

Patient Access to Health Data

Anil Sethi and Deven McGraw, chief executive officer and chief regulatory officer, respectively, of Ciitizen, discussed how its consumer health system helps Ciitizen customers—patients with cancer, autoimmune, or neurological diseases—securely collect, organize, and share their health data, including a patient's health records, imaging results, genomic data, functional status scores, and other documentation. By combining all of a patient's medical data into one easy-to-use summary, Ciitizen aims to provide both patients and clinicians a clear understanding of a patient's health and current care status. Sethi said Ciitizen improves on traditional EHR models in two ways: First, whereas EHRs are limited to the United States, Ciitizen is a global strategy; second, Ciitizen uses AI augmented by humans to code and compute medical data, which he said was more scalable than relying on human-generated data augmented by AI.

McGraw described Ciitizen's emphasis on patient privacy. She noted that Ciitizen will never share patient data in any form without patient consent, a commitment legally enforceable through the Federal Trade Commission. In addition, every user's data are protected through the California Confidentiality of Medical Information Act.[8] McGraw added that the Health

---

[7] For more information, see https://healthcaredelivery.cancer.gov/pro-ctcae (accessed June 7, 2020).

[8] For more information, see https://leginfo.legislature.ca.gov/faces/codes_displaySection.xhtml?sectionNum=56.10.&lawCode=CIV (accessed May 27, 2021).

Information Technology for Economic and Clinical Health (HITECH) Act[9] also requires disclosure of data breaches. McGraw stated that Ciitizen has adopted the most stringent industry-standard security safeguards and uses the most secure HIPAA-compliant cloud available. She called for a unified and robust federal privacy law to protect patient data, noting that the current patchwork system of rules and regulations impedes adoption of digital health technologies.

Dave Dubin, co-founder of the patient advocacy organization AliveAndKickn,[10] noted that patients like himself worry about protecting their health data, but also frequently need to transfer data among multiple clinicians and are often eager to share data for research purposes, with the goal of improving treatment for their condition. His registry, AliveAndKickn, collects data from patients with Lynch syndrome, the most common cause of hereditary colorectal cancer. By bringing these data together in a single clearinghouse, the organization can offer researchers access to large data sets and can help to match patients with relevant clinical trials.

Clinician-Oriented Technologies

Amid growing pressure to improve value in cancer care, Shulman said that digital tools present an opportunity to improve the quality of care while also improving efficiencies in care delivery. Several speakers described examples of clinician-oriented technologies designed to augment clinical decision making and streamline clinical workflows for improved cancer care delivery.

Machine Learning in Cancer Imaging and Pathology

Two speakers highlighted examples of tools that leverage ML for cancer pathology and imaging. Thomas Fuchs, founder of Paige.AI and director of computational pathology at Memorial Sloan Kettering Cancer Center (MSKCC), described several challenges in the field of cancer pathology: First, the complexity of cancer diagnosis is increasing, particularly with expanding molecular characterization of tumors. In addition, there are concerns about the workforce capacity limitations for pathologists, especially given the growing incidence of cancer due to the aging of the population. Fuchs posited that ML-based decision support systems in cancer pathology can help to address these challenges.

---

[9] For more information, see https://www.hhs.gov/hipaa/for-professionals/breach-notification/laws-regulations/final-rule-update/hitech/index.html (accessed May 27, 2021).

[10] See https://www.aliveandkickn.org (accessed June 14, 2021).

Fuchs said digital images of pathology slides can be used to develop ML algorithms to detect and grade cancers, and to help pathologists reach a diagnosis. Fuchs said that a major challenge for pathology algorithm development is the lack of digital pathology data sets for ML training, especially data sets that are generalizable to broad population groups. "Memorial [Sloan Kettering Cancer Center] started digitizing over 5 years ago. We now have approximately 1.5 million slides, which is 1.5 petabytes of data, and that allowed us to build models—for example, [an algorithm for] prostate cancer was based on 12,000 slides. At that scale, the hope is that you can build systems that represent reality and can be used in the clinic," said Fuchs.

Another challenge of ML algorithm development is annotating the slides for training the algorithm. Instead of time-intensive manual annotation of the digitized slides, Fuchs and his team used a new approach to train the algorithm directly from pathology reports (Campanella et al., 2019).

Fuchs posited that ML algorithms will play a key role in cancer diagnosis in the future, once they are rigorously validated and shown to be generalizable to broad populations and clinical practice settings, with appropriate regulatory review. Fuchs hopes that ML algorithms could help pathologists focus their efforts reviewing the more challenging cases, because pathologists can leverage the algorithm to make more straightforward calls about whether cancer is detected or not. He added that this could help democratize cancer pathology-specific expertise, typically available only at cancer centers or academic medical centers, and help improve diagnostic accuracy and precision within community oncology practice.

Sanjay Aneja, assistant professor of therapeutic radiology at the Yale School of Medicine, discussed how his team has applied deep learning to classify the presence of cancer within the lymph nodes of patients with head and neck cancer via diagnostic images (Kann et al., 2018, 2020). The team's ML model development pathway included starting with an important clinical question, finding and collecting appropriate data, comparing model candidates and selecting the best option, conducting external validation, and, following implementation, surveilling the results and conducting vulnerability studies to determine the model's effectiveness in clinical practice.

Aneja noted that preoperative identification of lymph node status via imaging could potentially reduce the need for surgical interventions and help determine whether there is extranodal extension[11] (ENE) of the cancer cells, which often requires adjuvant treatment escalation. The algorithm for lymph

---

[11] Extranodal extension occurs when cancer cells in a lymph node have broken through the capsule and spread into the surrounding tissue. See https://www.mypathologyreport.ca/extranodal-extension (accessed June 14, 2021).

node classification uses convolutional neural networks,[12] similar to the ML technology behind self-driving cars, image tagging, online banking, and other applications.

Aneja said the external validation of their model, using both local and national cohorts, demonstrated that the algorithm's classification of nodal involvement and ENE performed comparably to human classification, though further validation and vulnerability studies are needed prior to implementation. Aneja stressed that the intention is not for ML to replace radiologists; rather, ML tools can be incorporated to support their work, with the potential for performance gains, improved patient outcomes, and a reduced need for invasive surgeries.

Fuchs and Aneja were asked about the potential for integrated diagnostics—or the convergence of imaging, pathology, and health informatics—to improve cancer care. They responded that such multidisciplinary approaches would be beneficial, but would require data sets that are accessible across departments and institutions and are sufficiently large to produce clinically stable models. Aneja cautioned that careful attention is needed to avoid introducing bias when integrating multiple data sources.

Asked to reflect on research and policy needs to advance digital health, Aneja suggested that benchmarks be established for image analysis. He also suggested research to better understand and quantify performance loss. Specifically, he said efforts need to be placed on identifying clinical scenarios where algorithms perform significantly worse than human performance or whether algorithms have the same accuracy across all patient populations. Fuchs agreed, and noted that algorithms, however flawed, may be correctable in ways that human performance is not.

Fuchs also suggested that studies investigating ML in pathology should be broadened to include data representing diverse geographic areas, populations, and types of laboratories. He noted the challenge and expense of seeking FDA approval for diagnostic algorithms, but said it is imperative that these tools are validated and generalizable among broad contexts of use. While ML approaches will not necessarily reduce pathologists' growing workload, he noted that they have the potential to enhance care because they are able to detect patterns that may not be as evident to the human eye. These methods could also have a global benefit: many countries lack a sufficient pathology workforce, and ML-based tools could potentially enable nurses or medical technicians to take on some of this work, he added.

---

[12] In deep learning, a convolutional neural network is a class of deep neural network (a computer system modeled on the human brain and nervous system), most commonly applied to analyze visual imagery.

Informing Patient–Clinician Communication

Ravi Parikh, assistant professor in the Department of Medical Ethics and Health Policy and Medicine at the University of Pennsylvania and staff physician at the Corporal Michael J. Crescenz VA Medical Center, discussed the use of predictive analytics[13]—a technique long used by companies like Amazon and Netflix—to mine EHR data to inform and guide serious illness communication. Parikh said that early conversations about a patient's quality-of-life goals can help ensure that a cancer treatment plan is consistent with the patient's values, goals, and preferences, and avoids treatment with a low probability of benefit (Bernacki et al., 2019). Parikh said that University of Pennsylvania medical team members are trained to use the Serious Illness Conversation Guide to elicit patient preferences (Ariadne Labs: A Joint Center for Health Systems Innovation, 2017), but EHR documentation suggested this guide is underutilized. To address this gap, Parikh's team developed an ML-based classifier to help identify which patients may benefit from having serious illness conversations with their clinicians because they are at high risk for needing end-of-life care in the near future. The team integrated multiple sources of structured data to develop an algorithm with the goal of predicting which patients are at risk of dying within 6 months (Parikh et al., 2019b).

Parikh said a prospective validation study of the algorithm found that it accurately predicted the risk of short-term mortality (Manz et al., 2020a). Using the classifier, approximately 60 percent of the patients in the validation study were deemed appropriate to hold a serious illness conversation in the following week. Clinicians were then prompted to initiate these conversations in three ways: They received an email summarizing how often they held serious illness conversations compared to their peers; they were provided with a list of their patients who had been identified as high risk; and they were sent a text reminder (with the option to opt out) on days when patients with a high risk of dying within 6 months were scheduled for clinic visits. After these interventions, Parikh and his team found a three-fold increase in the use of serious illness conversations, and also found unexpected benefit—a spillover effect of better patient–clinician communication among all patients (Manz et al., 2020b). Parikh noted that clinicians were largely receptive to the tool, which he attributed to the involvement of clinicians in its development, its seamless workflow integration, and the potential to reduce clinician burden.

Parikh stressed that the actual intervention—the downstream care that is triggered by use of the classifier—is more important than the algorithm

---

[13] Predictive analytics is "the use of data, statistical algorithms and machine learning techniques to identify the likelihood of future outcomes based on historical data." See https://www.sas.com/en_us/insights/analytics/predictive-analytics.html (accessed May 29, 2021).

itself; for predictive analytics to improve care, he said they need to be coupled with an effective intervention. In this case, it was not the algorithm that changed clinician behavior, it was the intervention—the email and text—that prompted clinicians to initiate serious illness conversations. In addition, he emphasized that algorithms should be subject to rigorous evaluation—similar to how drugs and diagnostics are evaluated—prior to clinical implementation.

HEALTH DATA ACCESS AND USE

A number of workshop speakers said that health data from EHRs and other sources hold enormous potential to advance cancer research and to improve cancer care and patient outcomes. Researchers, clinicians, and technology developers are exploring the opportunities—and pitfalls—of accessing, integrating, and using health data in a variety of research and clinical contexts.

Leveraging Electronic Health Records and Artificial Intelligence to Improve Cancer Care

Two speakers focused on opportunities to leverage EHR data to bridge the divide between cancer research and cancer care: Neal Meropol, vice president and head of Medical and Scientific Affairs at Flatiron Health, and Allison Kurian, professor of medicine, epidemiology, and population health at the Stanford University School of Medicine and director of the Stanford Women's Clinical Cancer Genetics Program.

Meropol noted that while clinical trials are considered the gold standard for oncology evidence generation, they also have a number of drawbacks. They are expensive, and the long time it can take to initiate, recruit, and conduct a clinical trial may make the trial results less applicable to current practice, because of the rapid changes to the standard of care in oncology practice. In addition, clinical trials often fail to recruit participants who are representative of the overall patient population. He and Kurian discussed how using data-rich EHRs can help overcome some of these challenges to improve the evidence base for cancer care.

Meropol described how research using EHR data can fill critical evidence gaps in oncology. In addition to leveraging retrospective EHR data to generate high-quality evidence for new cancer insights and therapeutics, tapping into EHR data can help researchers define more relevant clinical trial inclusion criteria and also proactively identify patients who are eligible for clinical trials, potentially improving participant diversity and representation. Furthermore, the high-quality systems established for the collection, processing, and aggregation of EHR data, could also serve as an infrastructure for efficient data collection in prospective clinical trials. Meropol added that Flatiron Health collaborated on an examination of relationship between patient-reported quality of life data, and patient outcomes (Kerrigan et al., 2020), and is considering how its oncology EHRs could integrate ePRO data and how to effectively present these data to oncologists. There is mounting evidence and growing demand for using PRO data in research and cancer care, and these data need to be accessible, he said. Meropol also noted that FDA has allowed real-world health information to inform regulatory decision making, and EHRs are a critical source of these data.

He shared several examples of how researchers use Flatiron Health's EHR data to advance cancer research, including using de-identified EHR data for observational research in patients with non-small-cell lung cancer (Khozin et al., 2019); incorporating real-world data into the design of an algorithm to match patients with clinical trials (Kirshner et al., 2020); and assessing the impact of an FDA drug labeling change on treatment for patients with bladder cancer (Parikh et al., 2019a). Meropol noted that EHR data can also be leveraged to understand practice changes in the context of the COVID-19 pandemic, including the impact of the rapid increase in telemedicine visits and a decrease in in-person visits in 2020 (Green, 2020), suggesting an unprecedented opportunity to decentralize clinical trials and create a platform for a learning health system[14] that incorporates digital health data.

Kurian described the Oncoshare Project,[15] which integrates EHR data from two health care systems serving the San Francisco Bay area—Stanford University Medical Center, an academic tertiary care system, and Palo Alto Medical Foundation, a community-based system—along with data from the California Cancer Registry and genomic data from outside laboratories. Kurian noted that cancer data are currently fragmented across different data systems:

- Registries include data on patient demographics and survival, but contain limited information on diagnostic testing and treatment.
- EHRs contain a vast amount of clinical information, but often in unstructured text, making it difficult to mine and integrate with other data sources.
- Laboratory test results are also not integrated in EHRs.

---

[14] "A learning health care system is one in which science, informatics, incentives, and culture are aligned for continuous improvement, innovation, and equity—with best practices and discovery seamlessly embedded in the delivery process, individuals and families active participants in all elements, and new knowledge generated as an integral by-product of the delivery experience." See https://nam.edu/programs/value-science-driven-health-care (accessed June 17, 2021).

[15] See https://med.stanford.edu/oncoshare.html (accessed June 14, 2021).

The goal of the Oncoshare Project is to create a comprehensive data source to facilitate quality improvement and improve patient care. For example, as of July 2020, Oncoshare held anonymized, aggregated data from more than 28,000 patients with breast cancer.

Using data from the Oncoshare Project, Kurian and her team identified unwarranted variations in care among patients receiving care at both health care systems (Afghahi et al., 2016; Kurian et al., 2014). She said these patients who sought care at both systems had a higher number of invasive surgeries, greater use of imaging, and more treatment with chemotherapy and radiation therapy, yet there was no evidence of a benefit in survival among patients with higher utilization. Researchers have also used Oncoshare to discover new biomarkers associated with immune function and survival (e.g., lymphocyte count in aggressive triple-negative breast cancer) (Afghahi et al., 2018).

Thus far, the project's primary data source has been EHRs. Kurian noted that it remains difficult to access and integrate genomic data because they typically must be retrieved from laboratory PDFs. In the future, Kurian said Oncoshare plans to integrate tumor sequencing, imaging, and patient-reported data. In addition, the team plans to scale Oncoshare and validate its approach via national and international partnerships, including integration with the national Surveillance, Epidemiology, and End Results (SEER) program. Kurian identified scaling and real-time data integration as key priorities for enhancing the use of ML in digital health applications.

To further leverage data-rich EHRs and bridge health technology, clinical research, and patient care, Meropol stressed the need for common data models, strong data standards, shared interoperability elements, transparent regulatory requirements, and adherence to ethical principles. While it is important to collaborate with regulators, data organizers, technology developers, clinicians, and researchers, he said it is crucial for developers to listen to patients to ensure that products resonate with them; any health technology should be patient centered. Payer involvement is also key to creating appropriate incentives for users to adopt health technologies.

Using Artificial Intelligence to Improve Care Delivery

Sibel Blau, medical director of hematology-oncology at Northwest Medical Specialties and president and chief executive officer of the Quality Cancer Care Alliance Network, discussed how ML and AI technologies can be leveraged to improve care delivery, describing her organization's use of the predictive analytics tool Jvion.[16] Blau said that Northwest Medical Specialties is an

---

[16] For more information, see https://jvion.com (accessed June 7, 2021).

independent community oncology practice and research center that provides value-based care with continual data-driven practice innovations to improve efficiency, risk management, and outcomes. Jvion is an AI tool that analyzes clinical, socioeconomic, and demographic data to identify patients who may be at risk for adverse outcomes (e.g., metrics include 30-day mortality, 30-day pain management, and 30-day emergency department visits) and makes recommendations for actionable interventions to address these risk factors.

Northwest Medical Specialties customized the commercial Jvion product by defining key outcomes of concern (e.g., risk of emergency department visit within 30 days) and developing a workflow to address each outcome. They then incorporated EHR data into each workflow and added data on clinical and socioeconomic risk factors. The system used these data to generate individual patient-level risk profiles and to recommend interventions. Blau said that these recommendations have been instrumental in reducing clinician workloads, by relieving clinicians of exhaustive decision-making tasks and enabling them to focus on assembling patient care plans aimed at effectively and efficiently allocating limited resources while also improving outcomes.[17] Blau noted that this has helped improve clinician satisfaction.

Data analyses have also resulted in quality improvement efforts at Northwest Medical Specialties. For example, an analysis found that clinicians there recommended hospice care less often compared to other practices. In response, staff implemented advance care planning and palliative care visits for all patients diagnosed with advanced cancer, used AI to identify patients at high-risk of mortality, and implemented training in complex conversations. The practice has also improved other outcome metrics, including decreased patient utilization of the emergency department, a reduction in the number of patients experiencing a loss of physical functioning, an increase in the number of patients referred for treatment of depression, and a reduction in the number of patients reporting moderate or serious pain. In short, Blau stated that predictive analytics tied to interventions has led to improved patient outcomes and has become a key component of continual practice improvement.

Making Data Usable

The use of health data for research and practice improvements increasingly depends on the ability to access, understand, and combine data from different sources. These sources often span diverse organizations and jurisdictions. Several speakers addressed considerations related to data standards and policies to support the effective and efficient use of health data.

---

[17] For more information, see https://jvion.com/approach/clinical-implementation (accessed on July 7, 2021).

Data Governance and Access

Yann Joly, associate professor at the Faculty of Medicine, Department of Human Genetics, and research director of the Centre of Genomics and Policy at McGill University, offered an international perspective on data governance and access for digital health. He argued that making international health data accessible to clinicians will lead to better digital health tools. Digital health applications require vast training data sets; constraining data sets according to national borders therefore limits the effectiveness of these tools, especially for rare cancers. "The more data you get, the more data you fill into your tools and applications, the better they become," he said. "So, you need to think big, and that means you need to think not just local, but you need to think national and international." The International Cancer Genome Consortium, which includes data from more than 17,000 patients from 17 countries, is one model for sharing cancer data across borders. Joly noted that health data already travels beyond national borders during the process of internationally distributed cloud computing, which is required to analyze such massive data sets.

Joly said that international governance policies and standards are required to enable clinicians and researchers to use data safely and responsibly. He suggested such policies should incentivize data protection, address ethical issues, define liabilities and exclusions, and regulate digital health applications through a coherent and predictable global framework. In the absence of such a framework, he noted that data governance usually falls to international standards committees, which are limited to issuing nonbinding position statements that may not be adopted or integrated into law.

Joly outlined two strategies to achieve effective global data governance policies: national frameworks and laws can be retrospectively harmonized, broadened, or detailed to ensure alignment; or drafting new global laws. He pointed to two global health data organizations that could act as models: the Global Alliance for Genomics and Health (GA4GH)[18] and the Genetic Discrimination Observatory (GDO).[19] The GA4GH, made up of more than 500 international organizations, creates standards and guidelines to promote international digital health harmonization and interoperability. It has two cancer-related projects, the Beacon Project and the BRCA (BReast CAncer gene) Challenge. The Beacon Project aggregates members' genomic data from patients with cancer, enabling researchers to search the globe for particular genetic variants (Fiume et al., 2019). The BRCA Challenge is a plan to create an international database of BRCA variants to better understand BRCA muta-

---

[18] For more information, see https://www.ga4gh.org (accessed June 7, 2021).
[19] For more information, see https://gdo.global (accessed June 7, 2021).

tions and how they affect cancer risk. The GDO is a network of researchers and patients that seeks to strengthen international laws against genomic discrimination. The network allows patients to self-report their experiences, and policy makers can compare national approaches to promote harmonization.

Data Standards

Monica Bertagnolli, professor of surgery at Harvard Medical School and chief of the Division of Surgical Oncology at Brigham and Women's Hospital and the Dana-Farber Cancer Institute, outlined her work to create computable data standards across EHRs, an initiative called mCODE (Minimal Common Oncology Data Elements).[20] While EHRs contain valuable data with many potential applications for cancer research, inconsistencies in the types of information available and the way data are captured pose significant barriers. For example, data on patient tobacco use are recorded differently across EHRs (e.g., different categories can include nonsmoker, never smoked tobacco, ex-smoker, current smoker, unknown tobacco consumption, smokes tobacco daily, light smoker, occasional tobacco smoker, heavy smoker, etc.), which complicates efforts to use tobacco variables in analyses that incorporate EHR data from multiple institutions. In addition, some types of patient data are consistently available in EHRs, while others are only occasionally available and some are rarely recorded (see Table 1). Shulman added that current EHRs often cannot be used to determine basic information, such as whether a patient's cancer is metastatic. Bertagnolli noted that these data may exist within EHRs, but researchers lack the tools to retrieve them.

Bertagnolli said computable data standards are needed to integrate data sources and extract key information, which could enable the creation of widely applicable AI tools. The goal of mCODE is to develop and maintain data standards to achieve data interoperability and enable progress in clinical care quality initiatives, clinical research, and health care policy development. The CodeX (Common Oncology Data Elements eXtensions) community is a coalition of member organizations working collaboratively to integrate mCODE into existing and new applications using a Fast Healthcare Interoperability Resources (FHIR)[21] Implementation Guide. Bertagnolli stated that these standards will make critical health data accessible for AI retrieval and analysis, advancing progress in clinical care, clinical research, and health care policy.

The first version of mCODE has 73 data elements that are essential for oncology care. These elements and the standards that follow can be expanded

---

[20] See https://mcodeinitiative.org (accessed June 14, 2021).
[21] For additional information, see https://www.hl7.org/fhir (accessed June 8, 2021).

TABLE 1 Availability of Different Types of Data in Electronic Health Records

Generally Available	Sometimes Available	Generally Not Available
Diagnosis codes	Oral medications	Histology
Encounter codes	ER/PR/HER2 status	Genetic tests
Infused medication	Performance scores	Treatment intent
Laboratory tests	Hospice referral	Surgery
Smoking/Pain assessments	Staging (group and	Radiation therapy
Physical exam values	individual elements)	Imaging results
		Disease status (progressing, stable NED)

NOTE: ER = estrogen receptor; HER2 = human epidermal growth factor receptor 2; NED = no evidence of disease; PR = progesterone receptor.
SOURCE: Bertagnolli presentation, July 14, 2020.

on or adapted by researchers as needed. CodeX members develop and share best practices for implementing mCODE into EHRs, provide web-based mCODE training, and share clinical best practices for incorporating mCODE analyses. Bertagnolli noted that early mCODE applications show promise for enhancing patient care and the conduct of cancer clinical trials. For example, the ICAREdata collaboration used mCODE to obtain EHR data for clinical trial case reports. When mCODE was not able to provide necessary data, the CodeX community altered the code to prevent future gaps. Bertagnolli added that other research groups are testing use cases for mCODE to support clinical trials matching, patient registries, radiation oncology care coordination, clinical care pathways, and prior authorization to enable payment for care by insurers.

Brian Anderson, MITRE's chief digital health physician and the co-principal investigator of mCODE Standard Health Record, added that mCODE's common data model is critical to create a solid foundation for oncology data that enables effective use of digital health applications, enhances interoperability and workflows, and engages diverse participants. He stressed that patients and clinicians should be included in the design process for digital oncology applications. Patient voices cannot be overlooked, he said, and should guide ePRO and EHR design and data collection. Real-world data from ePROs and EHRs hold great potential to help design and launch clinical trials and support patient enrollment, and mCODE data standards could streamline the integration of this real-world data within clinical trials.

Bertagnolli expressed her hope that clinicians will welcome mCODE as an aid to clinical practice and not see it as a hindrance. However, optimizing clinical data for mCODE may require altering existing workflows to ensure data quality. Shulman noted that clinicians will be more likely to use digital health applications if those applications are able to free clinicians from low-value tasks. Blau commented that developing telehealth skills takes time and requires behavioral change, and recommended that EHRs include an AI component to quickly convert data into an interoperable form. Meropol agreed that easy-to-implement tools are important, provided they also produce high-quality data, and suggested that clinicians and payers collaborate on policies that establish and incentivize data quality standards.

POLICY CONSIDERATIONS

Many participants discussed how regulations and reimbursement influence digital health technology adoption in oncology research and care. They also examined the ethical and social implications of how technologies are designed, used, and governed.

Regulatory Considerations

Amy Abernethy, principal deputy commissioner of FDA, discussed how FDA approaches digital health applications for oncology, which digital interventions require FDA review, and the role that FDA can play in harnessing big data to benefit patients with cancer. She said that some—but not all—types of digital health applications require FDA clearance or approval prior to implementation in clinical practice. Abernethy noted that many digital health components that do not require FDA review are nonetheless of interest to the agency; for example, they may be important to the design of clinical trials that FDA may review for regulatory submissions. Abernethy stated that FDA is committed to supporting the development and implementation of digital tools for oncology: "Digital health is critical for learning health care systems and the continuous updating of medicine and our delivery of health care across time," Abernethy said. She noted that digital health is also critical to promoting patient-centered care in oncology—it is increasingly how clinicians collect PROs, communicate with their patients, and improve health care delivery.

Abernethy said that the fast pace of innovation across the landscape of digital health can make it challenging to determine whether a novel digital health application requires FDA review and she encouraged developers to consult with FDA's Center for Devices and Radiological Health (CDRH),[22] the entity that regulates medical devices. Abernethy noted that, broadly speaking,

---

[22] For more information, see https://www.fda.gov/about-fda/fda-organization/center-devices-and-radiological-health (accessed June 1, 2021).

if a clinician consults a digital health tool but makes the final treatment decision herself, FDA typically applies regulatory flexibility and allows the product to be used without FDA oversight. However, if a digital health tool interacts directly with a patient and makes recommendations, such as a chatbot triaging patient-reported symptoms, she said that application would typically require FDA review. She added that FDA does not regulate consumer devices such as fitness trackers because they are not considered medical products. However, if their use is for a medical purpose, such as monitoring for atrial fibrillation, they may require FDA review.

To keep pace with the constantly changing digital health landscape, Abernethy said FDA is now piloting a Pre-Certification Program, a regulatory pathway parallel to traditional device review that is designed specifically for the use of software as a medical device. "We acknowledge that the current regulatory pathways really aren't swift enough to accommodate solutions that are going to continuously change and adapt over time," Abernethy said. "The goal of the Pre-Certification pilot was to think about what the landscape would look like to approve a product that is anticipated to continuously change." The program has two major components: a review of the software development process to promote high standards and strict quality controls, and a schedule of continued evaluation to ensure that future updates also undergo review. Abernethy stressed that FDA is always available for specific questions and guidance. She encouraged workshop participants to review FDA's Digital Health Innovation Action Plan[23] and noted that the Digital Health Center of Excellence[24] serves as an additional resource.

Abernethy said that FDA's Oncology Center of Excellence has been a pioneer in incorporating real-world data and evidence into regulatory thinking. The 21st Century Cures Act[25] has also been critical, she said, by encouraging careful use of big data to facilitate decision making and improve patient care. COVID-19 is accelerating these efforts. "I think that 10-plus years of work is now accelerating very quickly in the context of COVID-19," Abernethy said. As an example, she pointed to the COVID-19 Evidence Accelerator,[26] which facilitates information exchange and collaboration to pose and address critical research questions. She noted that the initiative

---

[23] For more information, see https://www.fda.gov/media/106331/download (accessed June 1, 2021).

[24] For more information, see https://www.fda.gov/medical-devices/digital-health-center-excellence (accessed June 1, 2021).

[25] See https://www.fda.gov/regulatory-information/selected-amendments-fdc-act/21st-century-cures-act (accessed June 1, 2021).

[26] See https://evidenceaccelerator.org (accessed June 1, 2021).

follows the same model as an innovative oncology project[27] in which multiple groups collaborated to compare findings on immuno-oncology agents for lung cancer.

Abernethy noted that the COVID-19 Evidence Accelerator community is generating and using real-world and clinical trial data, demonstrating the benefits of teams collaborating around shared data under a single protocol with FDA guidance. Shulman agreed that this work can inform the medical community about agility, acceleration, and collaboration. Abernethy stressed that the medical community should continue to maintain high-quality standards, even at this new speed, to create trustworthy results. "We have to make sure that we are urgently doing work, but it is high-quality work and we're consistently cross-checking each other, and we're doing so in absolutely transparent ways," she said. Shulman agreed, noting that speed needs to be coupled with accountability to reduce the risk for error.

Legal Considerations

Kristen Rosati, partner at Coppersmith Brockelman PLC, discussed legal considerations in digital health, including data security and the complex laws governing privacy protections for patient health data. The Privacy Rule requires HIPAA-covered entities[28] to provide patients with access to their "designated record set," which includes their medical records, insurance claims, and other health information, and also gives patients the right to direct disclosure of these data to third parties. Rosati said that these rights are critical to facilitating care coordination, especially among patients with serious illnesses such as cancer, who may see multiple specialists to manage their care.

Two new regulations were recently adopted in the United States, with the aim of improving patients' access to their data and to facilitate data sharing. The first new regulation, which Rosati described as a paradigm shift, is The Office of the National Coordinator for Health Information Technology Interoperability and Information Blocking Rule.[29] Before this rule, health care organizations could only share patient data under specific circumstances set forth in the HIPAA Privacy Rule, and they were required to disclose data only to patients of the Department of Health and Human Services' Office for Civil Rights on request. Under the new rule, which was effective April 5,

---

[27] See https://friendsofcancerresearch.org/rwe (accessed June 17, 2021).

[28] HIPAA-covered entities are individuals, organizations, and agencies that are required to comply with the Privacy Rule. For more information, see https://www.hhs.gov/hipaa/for-professionals/covered-entities/index.html (accessed June 17, 2021).

[29] See https://www.healthit.gov/curesrule (accessed June 2, 2021).

2021,[30] health care organizations now must disclose patient health data when requested by any entity, unless data sharing is prohibited by law or if circumstances fall into one of eight exceptions in the rule. This rule applies to health care providers, health information exchanges or networks, and health IT developers of certified health information technology, including many digital health applications. The rule also contains new technical certifications for application programming interface (API[31])-enabled services. The rule carries up to a $1 million penalty for violations by health information exchanges or networks and health IT developers; the penalties for health care providers have not yet been defined.

A second new rule is the Interoperability and Patient Access Rule of the Centers for Medicare & Medicaid Services (CMS).[32] This rule requires government health plans to establish APIs for data sharing with third parties. However, Rosati cautioned that exact implementation details are unresolved, and patients currently are not protected by strong consumer data protection laws, and may unwittingly enroll in applications that could expose their data.

Rosati stated that these new rules add complexity to an already convoluted web of federal and state laws governing data sharing and patient privacy in the United States. "One of the primary problems with data sharing in the U.S. [...] is that we have this patchwork of laws that presently leaves a lot of information that's very important to patients unprotected," said Rosati. As an example of this complexity, the HIPAA Privacy Rule governs de-identification standards for health information, including genomic data, which is highly relevant for oncology, but there is no government guidance on whether genetic data can ever be considered de-identified. Health information is only protected if it is "individually identifiable," and the Office for Civil Rights has concluded that not all genetic information is individually identifiable. The common interpretation is that unless genetic information is accompanied by a HIPAA "identifier," genetic data is not protected by HIPAA. However, that interpretation may change as more genetic data are available in medical records and geneology databases that identify individuals associated with their genetic data. Moreover, the revised Common Rule has directed the agencies that enforce the Common Rule for federally funded research to issue guidance on whether

---

[30] In November 2020, compliance dates and timeframes were extended in response to the COVID-19 pandemic. For more information, see https://www.federalregister.gov/documents/2020/11/04/2020-24376/information-blocking-and-the-onc-health-it-certification-program-extension-of-compliance-dates-and (accessed June 8, 2021).

[31] An API is a software intermediary that allows two applications to talk to each other.

[32] See https://www.federalregister.gov/documents/2020/05/01/2020-05050/medicare-and-medicaid-programs-patient-protection-and-affordable-care-act-interoperability-and (accessed June 2, 2021).

any technologies (such as whole genome sequencing) should be treated as generating identifiable data. To operate amid these evolving regulations and technologies, practice responsible risk management, and protect patient data, Rosati suggested that cancer centers and researchers using genetic data should de-identify data via the expert determination method,[33] in a manner that aligns with federal, state, and international guidelines as applicable. She recommended that they also impose contractual requirements on third parties to prohibit data re-identification, restrict downstream disclosures, and ensure responsible data use.

Andrea Downing, president and co-founder of the Light Collective, described her experiences with this complex regulatory environment as a patient activist who carries a BRCA1[34] mutation. Downing said that patient rights and privacy protections are inadequate, especially outside of HIPAA-covered entities, which leaves individuals vulnerable to discrimination. When she was having difficulty navigating the health care system, she sought support from other members of the BRCA community, who shared deeply personal information within a closed group on social media. However, Downing raised concerns that the privacy settings could allow individuals outside of a closed group to have access to group members' information.[35] Arguing that health data deserves strict privacy controls, Downing suggested that all digital health applications should be subject to enforceable patient rights, a position she summarized as "no aggregation without representation."

Downing, McGraw, and Rosati noted that the protection of patient health data once it leaves the control of a HIPAA-covered entity is often unclear; outside of HIPAA, the patchwork of state and federal laws can leave many patients' data unprotected. Rosati argued for new, patient-centered, comprehensive federal data privacy laws that include genetic nondiscrimination protections. "We need a good federal data privacy law that doesn't apply just to HIPAA-covered entities," she said. "And then we need better discrimination laws to prevent the real discrimination that people experience [as a result

---

[33] Under the HIPAA Privacy Rule, there are two methods to achieve de-identification: creation of a safe harbor, in which 18 types of identifiers are removed from the data, or the expert determination method. In the latter, statistical or scientific principles are applied to render the data not individually identifiable, such that there is a very small likelihood that the anticipated recipient will be able to identify an individual from the data. See https://www.hhs.gov/hipaa/for-professionals/privacy/special-topics/de-identification/index.html#standard (accessed June 17, 2021).

[34] People who have certain mutations in a BRCA1 gene have a higher risk of breast, ovarian, prostate, and other types of cancer. See https://www.cancer.gov/publications/dictionaries/cancer-terms/def/brca1 (accessed June 2, 2021).

[35] See https://www.cnn.com/2020/02/29/health/andrea-downing-facebook-data-breach-wellness-trnd/index.html (accessed June 2, 2021).

of their] genetics." Rosati suggested that it may be possible to capitalize on bipartisan support for reform, partly driven by a desire among big technology companies to have consistent requirements across states. She added that California, which has privacy laws that apply to businesses even outside of the state, could also provide a model for a federal law. Joly argued that in addition to laws protecting patient privacy and genetic nondiscrimination, "I think we need also to think about administrative guidelines, standards of practice that are much more up to date, especially when you're talking about these digital technologies, because the scientific progress is so quick that you need to be able to change things [frequently]." He added it is also critical to react quickly when data breaches occur.

Elisabeth Belmont, corporate counsel for MaineHealth, noted that digital health technologies offer many benefits but also raise questions about their reliability, regulation, and how they affect malpractice risks. For example, in the case of remote monitoring devices, the data collected and used for clinical decision making could be unreliable if instructions are improperly followed or a recording is damaged. To mitigate this risk, she suggested that clinicians assess data quality or gather additional measurements to supplement clinical decision making. Belmont also noted that patient-generated data are not easily included in EHRs, and clinicians will need to adjust workflows to incorporate real-time patient data for patient care.

Belmont noted that remote digital telemetry applications used to monitor patient vital signs could potentially expose large numbers of patients to new risks, such as software errors. She added that there are currently no clear guidelines about disclosing AI errors or potential biases that could affect patient outcomes. She posited that malpractice law will also have to adapt to the new health technology landscape. For example, standards for negligence or liability may be more difficult to apply to algorithms that are continually changing. Courts can only use existing legal frameworks to define new technologies as "software" or "a device" and determine what regulations are applicable, she added, but these definitions are blurred when software is the device. For their part, it is important that clinicians heed their state licensing boards' rules, be consistent in their use of telehealth, follow in-person visit standards, and adequately document telehealth visits in EHRs, Belmont said. She also stressed the importance of flexibility—clinicians should be able and willing to arrange for in-person diagnosis or treatment if telehealth visits are inadequate for a patient's care.

Payment Models

Cathy J. Bradley, deputy director at the University of Colorado Cancer Center and associate dean for research at the Colorado School of Public

Health, discussed how payment policies—which can vary widely—affect the implementation of digital health applications. She noted that early digital health applications were primarily adopted in remote or underserved areas to improve access to care. Later, adoption was broadened to attempt to reduce the cost of care delivery. However, she said implementation was limited by a tangled web of inconsistent and opaque state reimbursement regulations and the absence of a federal reimbursement policy. Over the past 20 years, several major legislative acts have adjusted digital health reimbursements but the landscape remains complex, with technical innovation outpacing policy and legislation. She noted that this is especially true for oncology applications; for example, only two state Medicaid telehealth reimbursement policies specifically mention cancer, despite widespread implementation of telehealth services in oncology. Private payer policies evolved faster to adjust reimbursement, but still need to align their policies across the complex landscape of state laws.

Bradley described the rapid acceleration of the use of telehealth during the COVID-19 pandemic, with payers broadening coverage for approved services and platforms, to enable access to care while reducing the risk of infection. Telehealth adoption rates have varied across health systems, however. Bradley noted that teaching hospitals and clinicians within larger health care networks were better able to adapt to increased telehealth use, compared with public hospitals serving patients who have low incomes or are underinsured, for-profit hospitals, and hospitals subject to complex state licensing requirements. She noted that unless COVID-19-related reimbursement policies are extended, many patients will lose telehealth access when temporary policies expire.

Bradley argued that the post-COVID-19 era presents an opportunity to harmonize covered services and clinician reimbursement and to incentivize adoption of digital health technologies. "There's an opportunity now to create consistency and remove confusion in covered services and [reimbursement policies]," she said. "If our goal is to put telehealth infrastructure in place, remove restrictions for clinicians to practice across states, and incentivize through alternative payment models and payments for adoption, now is the time to put those in place permanently for patients." However, she cautioned that more evidence is needed to assess the impact on quality of care and patient outcomes, and the cost-effectiveness of telehealth.

Lara Strawbridge, who directs the Division of Ambulatory Payment Models at CMS's Center for Medicare & Medicaid Innovation, suggested that there are many options for creating payment models and said that models need to offer flexibility and autonomy to clinicians to provide the best patient care so that payers are not micromanaging decisions. Organizations like CMS, she said, will need to address several key questions to inform how digital health technologies such as ePROs are reimbursed and incorporated into oncology care going forward. First, given the critical need to engage patients and caregivers in decision making, it is important to determine how to incorporate ePRO data into oncology care workflows. This process is resource intensive and requires engagement of the full care team, especially considering that ePROs do not currently sync well with EHRs, she said. In addition, it is important to determine how best to evaluate ePROs for performance and reliability—qualities that are key in justifying reimbursement. Another question is whether AI tools can effectively integrate the numerous and different types of data streams to inform quality improvement efforts. Whereas some clinicians are clamoring for more data, having more data can be burdensome and overwhelming for clinicians unless it is presented appropriately, she said.

In addition to payment parity for telehealth and in-person clinical visits, Strawbridge said another potential policy option is the use of waivers to reimburse for telehealth services. It is also important to have appropriate guidance for determining when a visit should be done via telehealth versus in person, and how that affects treatment outcomes and existing health disparities. In a context of increasing emphasis on value-based care, a flexible payment model can allow clinicians to test alternatives and find solutions that work, she said.

Ethical Considerations

Digital health tools, like any other medical tool or digital technology, have important implications for individuals' privacy, data security, and safety. In addition, the way in which these tools are designed and implemented can perpetuate disparities that, even if unintentional, can cause real harm to patients. Several speakers examined the ethical considerations around digital health technologies.

Ethical Data Use

Nancy Kass, deputy director for public health and professor of bioethics and public health at Johns Hopkins University, highlighted ethical considerations for digital health applications, including transparency, consent, patient privacy, data security, data access and sharing, ownership and governance, justice, and benefits. She noted that organizations constantly make decisions about where health data go and what data will be de-identified, as well as who can access the data under what circumstances. Patients want assurance that their data are secure and they also want to know how the data are being shared, accessed, or protected, and for what purposes data are being used. For example, patient data could be used to inform care improvements within a health care system, for commercial gain, for independent research, or for a large federal research program such as the All of Us Research Program of the National Institutes of Health.[36] Each of these scenarios may raise different ethical obligations and concerns.

Kass stated that decisions about health data use and protections should be made transparent to patients. She stressed that consent for data use should require meaningful communication, not just blanket usage agreements rife with complex legal jargon. Patients should be informed about details of data usage, including whether data use will be disclosed, whether permission is needed before data can be used, and whether there a mechanism to opt out of data sharing. Kass added that patients should also be told if their data will only be used internally or if the data will be shared outside of an institution, and who will benefit from the data analysis. She noted that clarity around data ownership and governance lets patients know who is making decisions and whether they will have a say in the usage of their data.

Kass stated that clinicians who seek to use patients' health data with integrity should commit to transparency, ongoing engagement, and conducting studies that benefit patients who are traditionally underrepresented in research. From a justice and fairness perspective, it is key to consider whose data are used, what inferences can be drawn, and what biases may exist. Including patient participants in the decision-making process can improve transparency and responsiveness to patients' concerns and priorities, she noted. Integrity and trustworthiness also require that data users keep their commitments to patients; Kass emphasized that patients should be told immediately and meaningfully when these commitments are breached. In addition, she called for incentives and penalties to ensure that proper ethical protocols are followed.

Several participants discussed opportunities to facilitate patients' consent, and even compensation, for sharing their health data. Rosati pointed to the expense and logistical difficulty of seeking patients' consent in large-scale data sharing, noting that the requirement could hamper research. Instead, she suggested a community representative model, noting that broader financial incentives and shared decision making may be more effective than a model based on individual transactions. Downing, noting a trend in this direction, suggested the next step is to create a community-based, data-sharing model for patients with cancer that supports better understanding within the health care system of fair representation, implicit bias, and other complexities. Kass agreed that community benefits should outweigh individual benefits. She also emphasized that participant engagement is the key to understanding a digital application's value to patients, which developers can then use to enhance its effectiveness. A seal of approval, commending an application for its data privacy or community focus, could also help patients decide whether or not to participate, she suggested.

---

[36] For more information, see https://allofus.nih.gov (accessed June 14, 2021).

Addressing Racial Disparities in Oncology Care and Digital Health

Kadija Ferryman, industry assistant professor at New York University's Tandon School of Engineering, discussed racial disparities and racism in oncology care and digital health applications.[37] She noted that racial minority populations in the United States are more likely to be diagnosed with and die from cancer. For example, Black women are more likely than White women to die from breast cancer (Stringer-Reasor et al., 2021), not primarily because of biological differences but because of social factors like racism and implicit bias, Ferryman said. She added that the development and implementation of digital health technologies can also perpetuate racial biases. For example, a lack of visual representation of people of color in digital health tools may support the false belief that people of color are less at risk from cancer (Allicock et al., 2013). Ferryman noted that this lack of representation belies the true risk—people of color have higher incidence and worse outcomes for many types of cancer.

Ferryman noted that data sets used to train AI tools are less likely to include people of color, which can reduce the accuracy of AI tools among these populations (Lashbrook, 2018). Ferryman said that a grassroots social media movement, Brown Skin Matters, aims to address the problem of inadequate representation of dark skin with dermatological conditions for clinician and AI training. She said another source of racial bias is race-based adjustments to cancer risk calculations. These adjustments may be integrated into algorithms used in health care, and thus be invisible to clinicians who use the output of an algorithm for clinical decision making (Vyas et al., 2020). Ferryman noted that a frequently used "race correction" falsely lowers the expected cancer risk for people of color, leading to decreased surveillance, delayed diagnosis, and poorer outcomes (Vyas et al., 2020). Some health systems have removed racial corrections from their digital tools, but they may still remain in many currently used tools, because the embedded algorithms are not publicly shared.

To address racism in oncology care and avoid further exacerbating health disparities, Ferryman urged clinicians to prioritize health equity and ensure that data are not used to perpetuate race-based advantages (Ferryman and Winn, 2018). She said this same recommendation applies to digital oncology applications, which, Ferryman argued, should prominently feature people of color, use training data that are representative of diverse patient populations and evaluated for bias, and prioritize equity to address health disparities.

---

[37] See also *Applying Big Data to Address the Social Determinants of Health in Oncology: Proceedings of a Workshop* (NASEM, 2020a) and *Improving Cancer Diagnosis and Care: Clinical Application of Computational Methods in Precision Oncology: Proceedings of a Workshop* (NASEM, 2019).

"We've seen examples of where not having that background knowledge [on health disparities] at the outset has cascading effects later on," she said. "The earlier that you can build in some of these 'accountability practices,' the better the product will be downstream and the more robust the overall ecosystem of accountability will be." When race and racism are acknowledged at every level, she said, these tools will be able to promote equity and mitigate, not worsen, disparities.

Cleo Samuel-Ryals, associate professor at the University of North Carolina at Chapel Hill, asked how to ensure that AI developers consider equity in their algorithms. Ferryman replied that digital health regulations should require nondiscrimination in AI and ML and have strong enforcement. In addition, she suggested that FDA should include equity in its evaluations; industry should develop good practices and strong accountability; and companies should maintain awareness of health disparities, data representation, and implicit bias throughout the development process to reduce downstream inequities. Holding developers accountable, having robust and comprehensive policies, and highlighting equity issues in multiple places will lead to better AI tools, she said.

REFLECTIONS AND SUGGESTIONS

Throughout the workshop, participants discussed examples of digital health tools in action; examined the opportunities for digital health to advance cancer treatment, improve care delivery, and support oncology research; and identified critical questions, needs, and potential challenges as the oncology field moves toward their broader adoption.

Reflecting on these themes, Shulman underscored the need for digital health applications in oncology to facilitate patient–clinician communication and patients' engagement in their care. He stressed that involving patients and clinicians in the design process for digital health applications is essential to achieving these benefits. Peterson agreed, and said that successful patient-facing applications should keep the perspectives of patients, clinicians, and payers at the forefront throughout the entire development life cycle of the tool or technology. She urged developers to be responsive to evolving circumstances affecting the use of their technologies and to continually revisit and address patient, caregiver, and clinician needs.

Alicyn Campbell, head of digital health, oncology research and development, at AstraZeneca, said that digital tools have had the opportunity to improve cancer care and facilitate social distancing during the COVID-19 pandemic. In addition, she suggested that contributing data digitally may help patients feel more like equals in the patient–clinician dynamic. She urged developers to prioritize clinician and patient input, in order to facilitate integration of the digital technologies into the clinical workflow and to maximize usability and impact. Levy agreed, adding that technology adoption is dependent on clinicians valuing the data these tools provide.

Campbell added that patient involvement at every step of the development process enhances relevance and usefulness, which can also facilitate adoption, adding that it is especially important for digital health tools to be bidirectional—both eliciting information from and providing feedback to patients. Basch agreed that immediate and meaningful bidirectional feedback is important, and also added that successful patient-facing digital health tools share several other elements: patients are told from the beginning that this is an essential part of their care, technology use is well integrated into the care workflow, and nonengagement is monitored and gently addressed. He urged those developing and implementing digital health technologies to maintain a strong focus on health equity.

Many participants highlighted how remote monitoring, ePROs, telehealth, and EHRs offer vast and potentially powerful data sources for clinical research and improvements to care delivery. At the same time, many speakers emphasized that research is critical for understanding the utility of digital applications in different contexts. "Research really needs to be key in all of this. I think that we can't make assumptions about which digital applications are beneficial or not," Shulman said.

Campbell and Levy stressed that ensuring adequate reimbursement will be critical for the wide adoption of digital health tools in oncology practice. Campbell noted that, prior to the temporary changes in reimbursement made during the COVID-19 pandemic, many digital health companies had limited avenues for reimbursement. She stated that this failure to reimburse for digital health tools is a disservice to patients and clinicians, and suggested that novel reimbursement strategies will be key to incentivizing innovation.

Many participants highlighted ethical, legal, and safety considerations to ensure the safe and effective development of digital health tools in oncology. Shulman said that researchers need to be transparent about the purposes of data acquisition, aggregation, use and to honor promises made to patients. In addition, he said the complexity of the digital health landscape makes it especially important to ensure effective validation processes that take into account representation of different populations and the potential for bias, so that digital health tools do not exacerbate existing health disparities.

While oncology research and care have often been slow to change (due in part to their regulatory and financial complexities), Shulman said changes made in response to the COVID-19 pandemic have demonstrated that rapid change is possible, and he urged the oncology community to use this opportunity to advance digital health tools and technologies. Shulman stressed that a national push is needed from the entire oncology community to promote a better, evidence-based, patient-centered system of care delivery and research.

"We need national will from our patients, from our clinicians, from the regulators, and from the payers, to find a better path forward," he said.

REFERENCES

Afghahi, A., M. Mathur, C. A. Thompson, A. Mitani, J. Rigdon, M. Desai, P. P. Yu, M. A. de Bruin, T. Seto, C. Olson, P. Kenkare, S. L. Gomez, A. K. Das, H. S. Luft, G. W. Sledge, Jr., A. P. Sing, and A. W. Kurian. 2016. Use of gene expression profiling and chemotherapy in early-stage breast cancer: A study of linked electronic medical records, cancer registry data, and genomic data across two health care systems. *Journal of Oncology Practice* 12(6):e697–e709.

Afghahi, A., N. Purington, S. S. Han, M. Desai, E. Pierson, M. B. Mathur, T. Seto, C. A. Thompson, J. Rigdon, M. L. Telli, S. S. Badve, C. N. Curtis, R. B. West, K. Horst, S. L. Gomez, J. M. Ford, G. W. Sledge, and A. W. Kurian. 2018. Higher absolute lymphocyte counts predict lower mortality from early-stage triple-negative breast cancer. *Clinical Cancer Research* 24(12):2851–2858.

Allicock, M., N. Graves, K. Gray, and M. A. Troester. 2013. African American women's perspectives on breast cancer: Implications for communicating risk of basal-like breast cancer. *Journal of Health Care for the Poor and Underserved* 24(2):753–767.

Ariadne Labs: A Joint Center for Health Systems Innovation. 2017. *Serious Illness Conversation Guide*, edited by Dana Farber Cancer Institute. Boston, MA: Ariadne Labs and Dana Farber Institute.

Barbera, L. C., R. Sutradhar, C. Earle, N. Mittmann, H. Seow, D. Howell, Q. Li, and T. Deva. 2019. The impact of routine ESAS use on overall survival: Results of a population-based retrospective matched cohort analysis. *Journal of Clinical Oncology* 37(15 Suppl):6509.

Basch, E. 2010. The missing voice of patients in drug-safety reporting. *The New England Journal of Medicine* 362(10):865–869.

Basch, E., A. M. Deal, M. G. Kris, H. I. Scher, C. A. Hudis, P. Sabbatini, L. Rogak, A. V. Bennett, A. C. Dueck, and T. M. Atkinson. 2016. Symptom monitoring with patient-reported outcomes during routine cancer treatment: A randomized controlled trial. *Journal of Clinical Oncology* 34(6):557.

Basch, E., A. M. Deal, A. C. Dueck, H. I. Scher, M. G. Kris, C. Hudis, and D. Schrag. 2017. Overall survival results of a trial assessing patient-reported outcomes for symptom monitoring during routine cancer treatment. *JAMA* 318(2):197–198.

Beg, M. S., A. Gupta, T. Stewart, and C. D. Rethorst. 2017. Promise of wearable physical activity monitors in oncology practice. *Journal of Oncology Practice* 13(2):82–89.

Bernacki, R., J. Paladino, B. A. Neville, M. Hutchings, J. Kavanagh, O. P. Geerse, J. Lakin, J. J. Sanders, K. Miller, S. Lipsitz, A. A. Gawande, and S. D. Block. 2019. Effect of the serious illness care program in outpatient oncology: A cluster randomized clinical trial. *JAMA Internal Medicine* 179(6):751–759.

Campanella, G., M. G. Hanna, L. Geneslaw, A. Miraflor, V. Werneck Krauss Silva, K. J. Busam, E. Brogi, V. E. Reuter, D. S. Klimstra, and T. J. Fuchs. 2019. Clinical-grade computational pathology using weakly supervised deep learning on whole slide images. *Nature Medicine* 25(8):1301–1309.

Denis, F., E. Basch, A. L. Septans, J. Bennouna, T. Urban, A. C. Dueck, and C. Letellier. 2019. Two-year survival comparing web-based symptom monitoring vs routine surveillance following treatment for lung cancer. *JAMA* 321(3):306–307.

Ferryman, K., and R. Winn. 2018. Artificial intelligence can entrench disparities—here's what we must do. *The Cancer Letter* 44(43).

Fiume, M., M. Cupak, S. Keenan, J. Rambla, S. de la Torre, S. O. M. Dyke, A. J. Brookes, K. Carey, D. Lloyd, P. Goodhand, M. Haeussler, M. Baudis, H. Stockinger, L. Dolman, I. Lappalainen, J. Tornroos, M. Linden, J. D. Spalding, S. Ur-Rehman, A. Page, P. Flicek, S. Sherry, D. Haussler, S. Varma, G. Saunders, and S. Scollen. 2019. Federated discovery and sharing of genomic data using beacons. *Nature Biotechnology* 37(3):220–224.

Green, B. 2020. An emerging story: What data tell us about the impact of COVID-19 in community oncology. *flatiron* (blog), April 14, 2020. https://flatiron.com/blog/impact-covid-community (accessed Janaury 6, 2020).

Gresham, G., A. E. Hendifar, B. Spiegel, E. Neeman, R. Tuli, B. Rimel, R. A. Figlin, C. L. Meinert, S. Piantadosi, and A. M. Shinde. 2018. Wearable activity monitors to assess performance status and predict clinical outcomes in advanced cancer patients. *NPJ Digital Medicine* 1(1):27.

Innominato, P., S. Komarzynski, A. Karaboué, A. Ulusakarya, M. Bouchahda, M. Haydar, R. Bossevot-Desmaris, M. Mocquery, V. Plessis, and F. Lévi. 2018. Home-based e-health platform for multidimensional telemonitoring of symptoms, body weight, sleep, and circadian activity: Relevance for chronomodulated administration of irinotecan, fluorouracil-leucovorin, and oxaliplatin at home—Results from a pilot study. *JCO Clinical Cancer Informatics* 2:1–15.

Kann, B. H., S. Aneja, G. V. Loganadane, J. R. Kelly, S. M. Smith, R. H. Decker, B. Y. James, H. S. Park, W. G. Yarbrough, and A. Malhotra. 2018. Pretreatment identification of head and neck cancer nodal metastasis and extranodal extension using deep learning neural networks. *Nature Scientific Reports* 8(1):1–11.

Kann, B. H., D. F. Hicks, S. Payabvash, A. Mahajan, J. Du, V. Gupta, H. S. Park, J. B. Yu, W. G. Yarbrough, and B. A. Burtness. 2020. Multi-institutional validation of deep learning for pretreatment identification of extranodal extension in head and neck squamous cell carcinoma. *Journal of Clinical Oncology* 38(12):1304–1311.

Kerrigan, K., S. B. Patel, B. Haaland, D. Ose, A. Weinberg Chalmers, T. Haydell, N. J. Meropol, and W. Akerley. 2020. Prognostic significance of patient-reported outcomes in cancer. *JCO Oncology Practice* 16(4):e313–e323.

Khozin, S., K. R. Carson, J. Zhi, M. Tucker, S. E. Lee, D. E. Light, M. D. Curtis, M. Bralic, I. Kaganman, A. Gossai, P. Hofmeister, A. Z. Torres, R. A. Miksad, G. M. Blumenthal, R. Pazdur, and A. P. Abernethy. 2019. Real-world outcomes of patients with metastatic non-small cell lung cancer treated with programmed cell death protein 1 inhibitors in the year following U.S. regulatory approval. *Oncologist* 24(5):648–656.

Kirshner, J. J., K. Cohn, S. Dunder, K. Donahue, M. Richey, P. Larson, L. Sutton, E. Siu, J. Donegan, Z. Chen, C. Nightingale, and J. Hamrick. 2020. An automated EHR-based tool for identification of patients (pts) with metastatic disease to facilitate clinical trial pt ascertainment. *Journal of Clinical Oncology* 38(15 Suppl):2051.

Kurian, A. W., A. Mitani, M. Desai, P. P. Yu, T. Seto, S. C. Weber, C. Olson, P. Kenkare, S. L. Gomez, M. A. de Bruin, K. Horst, J. Belkora, S. G. May, D. L. Frosch, D. W. Blayney, H. S. Luft, and A. K. Das. 2014. Breast cancer treatment across health care systems: Linking electronic medical records and state registry data to enable outcomes research. *Cancer* 120(1):103–111.

Lashbrook, A. 2018. AI-driven dermatology could leave dark-skinned patients behind. *The Atlantic*, August 16, 2018. https://www.theatlantic.com/health/archive/2018/08/machine-learning-dermatology-skin-color/567619 (accessed June 6, 2021).

Manz, C., C. Chivers, M. Liu, S. B. Regli, S. Changolkar, C. N. Evans, C. A. Rareshide, M. Draugelis, J. Braun, and A. S. Navathe. 2020a. Prospective validation of a machine learning algorithm to predict short-term mortality among outpatients with cancer. *Journal of Clinical Oncology* 38(15):2009.

Manz, C., R. B. Parikh, C. N. Evans, C. Chivers, S. B. Regli, S. Changolkar, J. E. Bekelman, D. Small, C. A. L. Rareshide, N. O'Connor, L. M. Schuchter, L. N. Shulman, and M. S. Patel. 2020b. Effect of integrating machine learning mortality estimates with behavioral nudges to increase serious illness conversions among patients with cancer: A stepped-wedge cluster randomized trial. *Journal of Clinical Oncology* 38(15 Suppl):12002.

Marra, C., J. L. Chen, A. Coravos, and A. D. Stern. 2020. Quantifying the use of connected digital products in clinical research. *NPJ Digital Medicine* 3(1):1–5.

NASEM (National Academies of Sciences, Engineering, and Medicine). 2019. *Improving cancer diagnosis and care: Clinical application of computational methods in precision oncology: Proceedings of a workshop*. Washington, DC: The National Academies Press.

NASEM. 2020a. *Applying big data to address the social determinants of health in oncology: Proceedings of a workshop*. Washington, DC: The National Academies Press.

NASEM. 2020b. *The role of digital health technologies in drug development: Proceedings of a workshop*. Washington, DC: The National Academies Press.

Panagiotou, O. A., L. H. Högg, H. Hricak, S. N. Khleif, M. A. Levy, D. Magnus, M. J. Murphy, B. Patel, R. A. Winn, S. J. Nass, C. Gatsonis, and C. R. Cogle. 2020. Clinical application of computational methods in precision oncology: A review. *JAMA Oncology* 6(8):1282–1286. PMID: 32407443.

Parikh, R. B., B. J. S. Adamson, S. Khozin, M. D. Galsky, S. S. Baxi, A. Cohen, and R. Mamtani. 2019a. Association between FDA label restriction and immunotherapy and chemotherapy use in bladder cancer. *JAMA* 322(12):1209–1211.

Parikh, R. B., C. Manz, C. Chivers, S. H. Regli, J. Braun, M. E. Draugelis, L. M. Schuchter, L. N. Shulman, A. S. Navathe, and M. S. Patel. 2019b. Machine learning approaches to predict 6-month mortality among patients with cancer. *JAMA Network Open* 2(10):e1915997.

Peterson, S. K., E. H. Shinn, K. Basen-Engquist, W. Demark-Wahnefried, A. V. Prokhorov, C. Baru, I. H. Krueger, E. Farcas, P. Rios, and A. S. Garden. 2013. Identifying early dehydration risk with home-based sensors during radiation treatment: A feasibility study on patients with head and neck cancer. *Journal of the National Cancer Institute Monographs* 2013(47):162–168.

Stringer-Reasor, E. M., A. Elkhanany, K. Khoury, M. A. Simon, and L. A. Newman. 2021. Disparities in breast cancer associated with African American identity. *American Society of Clinical Oncology Educational Book*(41):e29–e46.

Tran, V.-T., C. Riveros, and P. Ravaud. 2019. Patients' views of wearable devices and AI in healthcare: Findings from the compare e-cohort. *NPJ Digital Medicine* 2(1):1–8.

Upadhaya, S., J. X. Yu, C. Oliva, M. Hooton, J. Hodge, and V. M. Hubbard-Lucey. 2020. Impact of COVID-19 on oncology clinical trials. *Nature Reviews. Drug Discovery* 19(6):376–377.

Vyas, D. A., L. G. Eisenstein, and D. S. Jones. 2020. Hidden in plain sight—Reconsidering the use of race correction in clinical algorithms. *The New England Journal of Medicine* 383(9):874–882.

Wright, A. A., N. Raman, P. Staples, S. Schonholz, A. Cronin, K. Carlson, N. L. Keating, and J.-P. Onnela. 2018. The HOPE pilot study: Harnessing patient-reported outcomes and biometric data to enhance cancer care. *JCO Clinical Cancer Informatics* 2:1–12.

Appendix A

Statement of Task

A planning committee of the National Academies of Sciences, Engineering, and Medicine will plan and host a 1.5-day public workshop that will examine opportunities and challenges, including validation, data security, and patient privacy issues, for the use of digital health applications in oncology. The workshop will feature invited presentations and panel discussions on topics such as:

- An overview of existing and emerging digital health applications and the potential benefits and risks associated with their use.
- Strategies to validate digital health applications, regulate their use, and mitigate potential risks associated with their use.
- Strategies for protecting the security of data collected using digital health applications.
- Patient privacy considerations, especially given the potential for data linkage with data from other sources of personal information.
- Best practices and principles for access to and consent for the use of patient data generated by digital health applications.
- Ways to integrate patient-generated health data into electronic health records and clinical workflow.
- Lessons learned from other industries and/or countries that could inform digital health application development and use.

The planning committee will develop the agenda for the workshop sessions, select and invite speakers and discussants, and moderate the discussions. A proceedings of the presentations and discussions at the workshop will be prepared by a designated rapporteur in accordance with institutional guidelines.

Appendix B

Workshop Agenda

July 13, 2020

9:30 a.m.   **Welcome from the National Cancer Policy Forum and the Forum on Cyber Resilience**
- Lawrence Shulman, University of Pennsylvania
  Workshop Planning Committee Chair
- Fred Schneider, Cornell University
  Chair, Forum on Cyber Resilience

9:45 a.m.   **Session 1: Overview of Digital Health Applications in Oncology**
Moderator: Lawrence Shulman, University of Pennsylvania

Digital Health in Cancer
- Mia Levy, Rush University Medical Center

Keynote Presentation
COVID-19 and Oncology Digital Health: Food and Drug Administration Perspective
- Anand Shah, Food and Drug Administration

Panel Discussion

10:30 a.m.   **Break**

10:45 a.m. Session 2: Lightning Round Presentations: Exemplars of Novel Digital Health Applications
Moderators: Deborah Estrin, Cornell Tech; and Randall Oyer, Penn Medicine Lancaster General Health

Patient-Facing Digital Applications
- Sam Takvorian, University of Pennsylvania
- Andrea Pusic, Harvard Medical School
- Panel Discussion

Radiology and Pathology Digital Applications
- Thomas Fuchs, Memorial Sloan Kettering Cancer Center
- Sanjay Aneja, Yale University
- Panel Discussion

Research/Electronic Health Records/Databases
- Allison W. Kurian, Stanford University
- Ravi Parikh, University of Pennsylvania
- Panel Discussion

12:15 p.m. Break

1:00 p.m. Session 3A: Food and Drug Administration Vision and Priorities for Regulating Digital Health Applications—Q&A with Lawrence Shulman
- Amy Abernethy, Food and Drug Administration

1:35 p.m. Session 3B: Ethical, Security, Governance, and Payment Issues with Digital Health Applications in Oncology
Moderators: Deven McGraw, Ciitizen; and Bradley Malin, Vanderbilt University

Legal Considerations—Patient Privacy and Data Security
- Kristen Rosati, Coppersmith Brockelman PLC

Ethics and Digital Health: What Is the Purpose of a Digital Health System and What Must Be Its Ethical Commitments?
- Nancy E. Kass, Johns Hopkins University

Data Governance and Access: International Perspective
- Yann Joly, McGill University

Race Matters in Oncology Apps
- Kadija Ferryman, New York University Tandon School of Engineering

Payment Policy: Digital Health and Access
- Cathy J. Bradley, University of Colorado Cancer Center

Panel Discussion
Include speakers and
- Andrea Downing, The Light Collective

2:55 p.m. Break

3:05 p.m. Session 4: Patient-Facing Digital Technologies
Moderator: Karen Basen-Engquist, The University of Texas MD Anderson Cancer Center

Patient Access to Their Health Data, Storage, and Portability
- Anil Sethi and Deven McGraw, Ciitizen

Electronic Patient-Reported Outcomes as Digital Therapeutics
- Ethan Basch, University of North Carolina

Wearable, Mobile, and Remote Monitoring Technologies in Oncology: Current Evidence and Future Opportunities
- Susan Peterson, The University of Texas MD Anderson Cancer Center

Telehealth in Oncology: Learnings from the Rapid and Broad Implementation During the COVID-19 Pandemic
- Mia Levy, Rush University Medical Center

Panel Discussion
- Alicyn Campbell, AstraZeneca
- Dave Dubin, AliveAndKickn

4:15 p.m. Adjourn Day 1

July 14, 2020

9:00 a.m. **Cancer Medicine, Digital Health, and the COVID-19 Pandemic ... and After ...**
- Lawrence Shulman, University of Pennsylvania
  Workshop Planning Committee Chair

9:10 a.m. **Session 5: Opportunities to Improve Data Availability and Usage in Electronic Health Records and Large Databases**
Moderator: Lawrence Shulman, University of Pennsylvania

Leveraging Electronic Health Records to Narrow the Divide Between Research and Practice
- Neal Meropol, Flatiron Health

Minimal Common Oncology Data Elements (mCODE)
- Monica Bertagnolli, Dana-Farber Cancer Institute/ Brigham and Women's Cancer Center

Utilizing Data and Machine Learning to Change Predictive Analytics into Prescriptive Analytics
- Sibel Blau, Quality Cancer Care Alliance Network

Panel Discussion
Include speakers and:
- Brian Anderson, MITRE Corporation

10:15 a.m. Break

10:25 a.m. **Session 6: Panel Discussion: Participant Reactions and Recommendations for the Path Forward**
Moderator: Lisa Kennedy Sheldon, Oncology Nursing Society

Panelists (5 minutes each for introductory remarks)
- Elisabeth Belmont, MaineHealth
- Paul Kluetz, Food and Drug Administration
- Mia Levy, Rush University Medical Center
- Neal Meropol, Flatiron Health
- Susan Peterson, The University of Texas MD Anderson Cancer Center
- Lara Strawbridge, Centers for Medicare & Medicaid Services

Discussion

11:30 a.m.	**Workshop Wrap-Up** • Lawrence Shulman, University of Pennsylvania Workshop Planning Committee Chair
11:45 a.m.	**Adjourn**